THE PRACTICE IS THE PATH

THE
PRACTICE
IS THE
PATH

LESSONS AND REFLECTIONS ON
THE TRANSFORMATIVE POWER OF YOGA

Tias Little

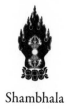

Shambhala

Shambhala Publications, Inc.
4720 Walnut Street
Boulder, Colorado 80301
www.shambhala.com

Cover art: LuckyStep/Shutterstock
Cover design: Daniel Urban-Brown and Kate E. White
Interior design: Greta D. Sibley

9 8 7 6 5 4 3 2 1

First Edition
Printed in the United States of America

∞ This edition is printed on acid-free paper that meets the
American National Standards Institute z39.48 Standard.
♲ This book is printed on 30% postconsumer recycled paper.
For more information please visit www.shambhala.com.
Shambhala Publications is distributed worldwide by
Penguin Random House, Inc., and its subsidiaries.

Library of Congress Cataloging-in-Publication Data
Names: Little, Tias, author.
Title: The practice is the path: lessons and reflections on
the transformative power of yoga/Tias Little.
Description: Boulder, Colorado: Shambhala, 2020. |
Includes bibliographical references.
Identifiers: LCCN 2019048509 | ISBN 9781611807370 (trade paperback)
Subjects: LCSH: Yoga.
Classification: LCC B132.Y6 l555 2020 | DDC 204/.36—dc23
LC record available at https://lccn.loc.gov/2019048509

To my father, H. Ganse Little Jr. (1932–2018),
professor of religion, Williams College, Massachusetts,
whose passion for learning inspired me to stride the
intricate trails of the psyche, soma, and spirit.

I dedicate this book to the myriad feet—bare feet,
booted feet, brown feet and white feet, small,
medium, and large in size—who have tread
this path before me, leaving behind a
trusted trail for me to follow.

Traveler, the path is your tracks

And nothing more.

Traveler, there is no path

The path is made by walking.

By walking you make a path

And turning, you look back

At a way you will never tread again

Traveler, there is no road

Only wakes in the sea.

—Antonio Machado, *There Is No Dream*

Contents

Introduction

NOT EVERYONE IN life finds a path that is meaningful and helps cure the spirit. Many never make it to the trailhead. More often, people end up moving through life in pursuit of the next best thing. Many, by default, end up on roads that lead them to strive for gain—making money, achieving popularity, and being successful. These roads have fast lanes, enabling people to move at greater speeds and achieve their goals in less time. Some end up in cul-de-sacs, confined by lives focused on pursuing pleasure and avoiding pain.

A path is different. On a path, you are meant to meander, to enjoy each footfall. Every ascent and descent is part of the journey. And there may be moments—days, weeks, and months—when you feel totally lost. A path is winding and circuitous and the experience of losing your way is part of the way. A path is wide enough only for footsteps. You cannot drive an RV equipped with a kitchen and flat-screen TV down it. By necessity, you must travel light.

Sometimes you find yourself on the path by happenstance, someone on a whim takes you there, or you look for it on the World Wide Web. It doesn't matter how you get there. What matters is that sure-footed, with shoulders back and heart lifted, you trust the pads of your feet.

The path I am speaking of is not a trail that cuts through canyons and meadows or crisscrosses the mountain. The path I am referring to is the Big Path, the Tao, the Way. It is a path that opens the lungs, fires the spirit, and awakens faith. It is the path of pilgrimage, one that leads straight to the heart of being.

This book is about being on that path—the Path. It is about an essential journey that begins the moment you hear the reverberation of an inner voice that says simply, "I must." It is about listening to the voice of yearning inside, despite the odds, and the many competing voices calling you back to familiar commutes along paved surfaces.

For many of us, there is one year in our lifetime that sets the stage for all other years, one year that shapes our destiny. For me, it was when I was seven, and a voice prompted me to delve into the caverns of my soul. A strange yearning took over my young and impressionable mind, a longing to explore the labyrinth of my inner self. It set me on a journey through many landscapes, teachers, instructions, and techniques. This voice, this spirit-whisperer, coaxed me on—at times gentle and merciful, and at other times fierce and uncompromising.

The trek has demanded every fiber of my being, and along the way, I have had to question the realities I assumed to be true. Through my teens and twenties, my internal navigation device worked erratically. I spent years traipsing off course, isolated in remote canyons and narrow tunnels. All too often I found myself stranded, having strayed from essential connections to myself and others. But despite years of disorientation and confusion, an inner longing, a hidden hunger, prompted me to persevere.

On a mountain path there can be many obstacles: mud, fallen trees, rocks, washed-out terrain. Yet the spiritual path is more arduous, for the obstacles are not external but internal. On my own path, I have had to contend with stumbling blocks that are essentially products of my own making. They include my urge toward perfection, a desire to be good, a tendency to push my way forward, restlessness, craving, and a fear of letting go. I believe these hindrances are common to many fellow seekers on the path, so I will attempt to address them in this book.

A path is made by the multitudes who have gone before us. Like river rock, smoothed and polished by the ongoing flow of water, the path has been worn by wayfarers on quests similar to yours and mine. Thus we do not have to carve out a new trail. At first, we must learn to follow. The intent to follow guides us away from the false notion that this is "my way." As we follow we take faith, and the path itself is the guru, the guide.

It is a godsend to find a path that enables the maturation of the soul. For me the path has been yoga, but any craft—such as acting, cooking, woodworking, or playing an instrument—may suffice to steer you into landscapes unimaginable. In this book I reflect on the changing horizons I have seen on the trail. I look back on the time I first embarked from the trailhead, the expectations I had of myself and the assumptions I held about the journey's end. I see now that what I thought was enlightenment was part of a greater delusion.

In the first half of the journey, we adhere to order, security, rote discipline. We are more inclined to live by the letter of the law rather than its spirit. We may impose strict boundaries on ourselves and be quick to judge others. Idealistic and moralistic, we may approach spirituality from the side of our small-minded self, eager to be liked, obtain approval and succeed. Out of a desire to gain a solid foothold within ourselves, we get attached to our systems, our techniques, our memorized verses, our badges and brands. In the beginning we need affirmation that we are making progress— success and security are paramount. We may overidentify with a style of practice, a sequence of poses, or a system of teachings. In the first half of my journey, I held strongly to the code of Ashtanga yoga, vegetarianism, and mantra. Initially, these foundational prac- tices provided important footholds that enabled me to climb. In the arduous migration of the soul, however, we all come to a crossroads where we must relinquish all title, rank, and name. This demands another kind of exodus, one that involves risk and surrender.

The first half of my climb lasted until the end of my thirties.

Several formative experiences prompted me to gain a more panoramic view of myself and insight into the heart of the yoga teachings. The first involved my forays into Zen and the Middle Way teachings of the Buddha. When I first encountered the Heart Sutra and the cryptic yet compelling instruction "Form is emptiness and emptiness is form," my very foundation rocked off its center. The second was by plummeting into the murky world of dreams. Through dreamwork I caught glimpses of the longing, fear, and urges that reside in the umbra of my psyche.

It is oftentimes a split, some traumatic moment, loss, or rupture that prompts us to break through the boundaries of our early practice. This can be threatening, painful, even shocking because we become so invested in the initial formulas that provide us with grounding and stability. Why on earth would it need to change? Yet in order to evolve, we must leave behind the strict order of the first half of practice and enter a new phase—one in which we realize the fragility and insubstantiality of the self. In the second half of the journey, we are made humble and stand in awe of the mystery. We step out of the shackles of shame and doubt and form a liaison with a force much greater than ourselves. This book is really for students who have made a practice for themselves in the first half of their journey.

In the beginning, the path is often defined by attitudes and beliefs that we bring to the mat. Within our connective tissues we hold a history—a personal narrative of thoughts, memories, and ideals. We may harbor inflated (or deflated) expectations of ourselves. Much is at stake, and a potentially crippling crisis arises.

Caught in the quandary of self, we struggle with feelings of pride or shame. There is anxiety and a gnawing apprehension: *Am I getting this right? Am I good enough? Am I worthy?*

Unbeknownst to ourselves, we each lug around a heavy pack stuffed with a longing for acceptance and a fear of rejection. At the beginning of the trail, and from a vantage point that is extremely limited, we equip ourselves with ideas and beliefs *about* the journey. In the beginning we make elaborate assumptions about the way we should be. The soul is yet to pass through the gates of fire, loneliness, and deep silence that build maturity and wisdom. We have yet to experience loss and suffering and to witness directly the beauty and fallibility of our own small, fragile selves.

When we first come to the mat, our beliefs may have been molded by an overarching religious structure that is wont to divide the world in two: right and wrong, good and bad, male and female, pure and sullied, true and false. Armed with fixed convictions, we unwittingly block the flow of the soul-self, which is fluid, shadowy, polymorphous, and full of a raw and wild energy. The enduring spirit of the soul-self is nonconforming.

At the beginning of a yoga path, we may simply wish to become sleeker, sexier, more efficient, or more powerful. We may have a burning desire to get away from where we are. Progress on the path typically becomes a kind of self-improvement project. We may use the practice as a means to escape either the pressures of work, our personal history, or the drone of our own thoughts. Because we are driven by self-interest, the path is inevitably narrow, and we can only see a few yards ahead.

These first years involve hardship. Physical hardship. We experience pain in our knees, back, and shoulders. In many instances, we seek out physical hardship through "power" practices that are strenuous and uncompromising. If we make it through the early trials of practice, the body and mind start to break open. We become less constricted and guarded, less myopic. The dimensions of the path widen, and we begin to see bigger and broader horizons. The path is no longer proscribed by our three-by-six sticky mat. From the vantage point of a more panoramic view, we become more available to others. In the flow of our daily lives we are more adaptable, more able to meet the demands of changing circumstances.

One of my Zen teachers would always ask, "How wide is your path?" Might we see in time that the path is everywhere? Might the way of our path, like the old Tao, include all things?

In this book, we will travel the path together, a path that enables us to see beyond the confines of our own perspective. Each vista on the path is inevitably circumscribed by the view we are afforded, just as we must experience the world from the limited standpoint of our own small selves. In the journey that lies ahead, we must leave behind the person we always thought we should be and travel, step by step, to where we are. There is really only one way to do this, for as we will see in the chapters ahead, the practice is the path.

—Tias Little
Santa Fe, New Mexico
August 2019

THE PRACTICE IS THE PATH

Empty before
You Begin

I TYPICALLY BEGIN my classes with *savasana* (corpse pose). I have students lie down on their backs and be still. I say, "Empty before you begin," encouraging them to let go of the pressures that may have accumulated during the day from work, driving, parenting, or simply trying to hold everything together. This is a way to slough off the burdens of the day and just be. While they are in savasana (I always use the Sanskrit for this pose since I find the English translation to be a misnomer), I encourage students to visualize strain or stress evaporating off their skin. It is an invitation to become an open vessel and become receptive to whatever may arise.

Empty before you begin is a most difficult practice. Typically the inbox of the mind is jammed with messages: private messages from family and loved ones, work-related messages that add to your task list, advertisements that goad you to acquire something you really don't need. It is only by emptying that we can become fully attentive and present. Empty before you begin is essentially a call to presence. Here at the start of this book, I implore you, reader, to empty before you begin—that is, to make yourself open and clear for each word on the page.

Ideally this process of emptying happens before you leave your home in the morning. When you actively let go at dawn (the ideal time for meditation practice), you prepare your mind and heart for the day. The key is to get up, take a pee, and go right to the cushion. Before checking your inbox or sending and receiving, sit in silence with a tall spine and lifted heart. At the threshold to your day, empty your thoughts, expectations, and management strategies. Just sit with a clear mind and a soft, open breath.

This can be an arduous task. Typically, if we are not careful, our minds get monopolized by the demands of the day. Deadlines and obligations engulf our attention. Insidious voices infiltrate our heads, and we find ourselves reviewing past conversations or rehearsing conversations to come. All too often when we wake up and open our eyes, a torrent of thought inundates our minds, like a dam breaking loose. When we learn to arrest the flood of thought, we rest in wide-open attention.

This process is something like opening an empty file, a new blank document, on a computer screen. Do not rush to fill your mind with text and images; allow it to be open space. This clear, uncluttered space of mind and heart is full of potential, full of possibility. The more you can rest in a spacious awareness in meditation, the more it will stay with you throughout the day, even in the midst of the hum and buzz of the daily round.

The mind can be like our home's garage after twenty or thirty years of residency—crammed full of old stuff, boxes stacked high toward the ceiling. We hold on to high school yearbooks, letters from long-lost mates, stuffed animals, old coins, memorabilia from vacations, photographs of moments in time. The storage space of the mind becomes cluttered. We are mind hoarders, holding on to people, events, and conversations. Like stuff heaped away in an attic or a garage, ideas, hopes, and fears pack our minds.

Through meditation, yoga, chanting, and prayer, we clean house. We sort through piles of personal history, troves of impressions, wants, and needs. In the beginning, this proves difficult, for it is hard to maneuver through the aisles of clutter. In sorting through the paraphernalia of our mind stuff, we get lost somewhere in the timeline of our personal history, in the narrative we have become.

When we get to the cushion and sit with a lifted spine, we must ask, *Out of all that I have accumulated, what really belongs?* We identify with our mind memorabilia, but is it really "me"? When we look long and hard over many sessions, we begin to realize that all the stuff we have compiled in our minds and hearts over the years is surplus. We come to realize that what we really need is to pare down, discard, and let go.

How do we let go in the midst of lives that are full to the brim? How do we learn not to hoard not only material possessions, but feelings, viewpoints, and ideals? This is where practice comes in. We learn bit by bit, breath by breath, to let go of who we think we are and who we think we ought to be. Yoga is as much a process of *un*learning as it is a path of learning. In the first years, our practice is like a raft, one that ferries us across the divide of self. It provides security and certitude and helps us travel. However, at some point, we must be willing to dismantle the very same raft that has carried us along. We give up the raft but keep the wisdom entrusted to us on the journey.

The process of unpacking and letting go begins in the body and involves a passage from outer to inner. For instance, at the beginning of yoga practice we do postures that stretch and loosen the superficial fascia, the outer covering of the body. This flexible layer of connective tissue, just under the skin, is responsible for determining our characteristic identity structure. Our exterior may be taut and constricted, or it may be lax and weak. In the first years of practice, we engage the outer musculature—the extrinsic muscles—such as the deltoids, traps, glutes, and hamstrings. In time (and this takes years), we open and activate the core musculature, the intrinsic muscles along the spine. Hatha yoga is a pilgrimage to the inner sanctum of the spine.

As we travel from outer to inner, we must shed or molt the outer layers of self. In this process, we are as delicate as new butterflies emerging from a chrysalis. At some point in the journey we realize that we are confined by our own outer cover, the cocoon-like structure of our exterior self. A short poem by the Japanese Zen poet Shuho captures this idea:

Cicada shell
little did I know
It was my life.[1]

A cicada is an obnoxious insect that makes ear-splitting clacking sounds in the summer heat. Maybe you recall finding its flimsy shell, its exoskeleton, like the hull of a small shrimp, clinging to a tree. The cicada nymph abandons its shell when it molts and emerges into adulthood. For hundreds of years in the poetic traditions of Asia, the cicada has been a metaphor for transience and spiritual metamorphosis. It is an analogy for the process of emerging, morphing from one state to another. The spiritual journey requires that when ready, we cast off the armoring that confines us so that an interior soul-self, tender and less constricted, can emerge.

Dropping the bulwark of armor is not easy, for it may have provided needed protection. Oftentimes the exoskeleton serves to protect us from the ghosts of our own past—from emotional hardship, trauma, and loss. It may provide a kind of refuge, one that we never received from family, school, friends, or lovers. Dismantling the armor is a necessary stage in the maturation of a yoga practice. It is tricky, for all too often we identify with our protective gear, given that our shell, at one time, was necessary to keep us safe. Thus we may not drop our shell all at once, but rather over days, months, even decades. We may discard our outer shell and then, feeling vulnerable and exposed, don the familiar protective covering. This can happen repeatedly: we remove our cover and put it on again. It takes time for the supple, open, tender inner self to have the courage and trust to be in the world without having to hide.

Some never make it out of their protective armor. By holding to rigid belief systems, people get stuck in chivalry, fear, and bigotry and defend their code of honor. Fundamentalist Christians, Hindus, Jews, or Muslims adhere to the binaries of *us versus them*, male or female, gay or straight, black or white, criminal or law-abiding, strong or weak—or as Dr. Seuss depicted so colorfully, the Star-Belly Sneetches versus the Plain-Belly Sneetches. Our beliefs about ourselves and the living world around us seep into our connective tissues—into the microbes of our gut, the organs of our heart and liver, and the synapses of our brain. "Belief becomes biology" wrote the author and educator Norman Cousins. Over time and with practice, we come to see the particular ways that our tissues get informed by convictions and assumptions.

Letting down our defense mechanisms while learning to let go is a difficult yet most essential practice. When we practice letting go, we loosen the fixed attitudes and beliefs that come to define us. For when the mind hardens around belief, it is a big fix! By letting go, we prepare to live an all-inclusive life, motivated by altruism, kindness, and tolerance. In raising children, being in relationship, aging, and dying, we actively let go. Ultimately, we must practice letting go in the midst of our daily rounds. In one day alone, we must let go five times, fifty times, ten thousand times. Living itself becomes a perpetual process of letting go.

This is not to suggest that we head straight for the checkout lane, abandon society, and move to Idaho to live in a concrete bunker. I don't suggest pulling the plug on your family, your livelihood, or your friends and neighbors. Rather the task is to interact with the world wholeheartedly, with passion and verve, while at the same time not becoming fixated or stuck. This requires a double movement, one that is difficult to do and requires simultaneously engaging and letting go.

We learn this double move in asana training when we learn to execute a pose. It is commonly called "opposing action," and it is worth learning. For instance, in a pose like half moon pose (*ardha chandrasana*), opposing action requires that the student press down through the heel of the standing foot while simultaneously drawing upward from the floor along the inner shin and knee. In other words, the student must move in two opposite directions at once. It is valuable to accomplish this "opposing action" somatically in concert with the psychological process of engaged letting go.

———

Breathing lies right at the heart of letting go. Each breath we take in and each breath we let out is practice in letting go. The breath itself becomes the guide, the guru, teaching us to empty and release. Also, we must learn to let go of thoughts, sensations, expectations, and judgments. With practice, every moment that arises is an opportunity to let go. The art of mindfulness is remembering to let go.

Over time we cultivate a willingness, a readiness, to let go. The longer we practice, the more we become predisposed to letting go.

Like training the body to ride a bike or the brain to memorize a poem, we train the "letting go muscle" in order to be free of malice, shame, ill will, and craving. We learn to let go of corrosive thinking so that it does not eat away our soft interior. Once established in the "memory" of letting go, we are prepared to be in the world without clinging to circumstances, people, or the changing tides of experience.

In this way, practice is preparation for how we live our lives. Yoga and meditation are all about alertness, readiness, having all systems go, so that we can engage in the world with open hearts and clear minds. The mettle of the spirit-warrior is to participate in the world without clinging. Like a soldier preparing for battle, hours and hours are spent training in the art of engaged letting go. This is the lesson of the warrior hero Arjuna. In the Bhagavad Gita, while rehearsing for the theater of war, Arjuna ironically equips himself with an attitude of yielding:

> Renouncing all objects of desire and willful purpose, completely restraining the senses and the mind, he should gradually relinquish all, holding firm to the *atma* (soul-self) he should rest empty of all thought.[2]

In premodern India, when yoga was being cultivated as a means to procure the spirit, both the warrior and priestly castes honed the will by concentrating the internal energies. By readying himself in the spirit of renunciation, the devout warrior prepared rigorously to live to the fullest without becoming attached to the outcome. The archetypal form of the seated Buddha captures this same spirit of preparedness and foresight. His enduring presence suggests readiness. The next time you look at a figure of the Buddha seated on a lotus pad, eyes cast downward and spine lifted, note his exquisite alertness and poise, anticipating everything to come, ready to let go.

We often imagine letting go to be a passive thing, akin to releasing our clasp on a balloon string. However, there is effort involved, sometimes referred to as "nonefforting effort." Right effort is cultivated in all of the martial arts, such as aikido, karate, tae kwan do, or jiujitsu. In the internal arts of tai chi, qigong, or yoga, right effort is the gateway to the subtle body. In chapter 4 we will investigate the perplexing practice of right effort in more detail.

There is a difference between active letting go and passive letting go. In savasana, when passively letting go, we typically fall asleep or check out. Active letting go is to observe frame by frame the process of emptying and releasing. Profound relaxation within the body facilitates greater concentration in meditation and helps cultivate a luminous field of awareness. When there is both physiological ease and psychological space, we yoke to a force much larger than ourselves.

In many regards, yoga is truly a preparation for death, the final letting go (an idea we will explore in chapter 9). When we empty before we begin, we are enacting a little death. We train by witnessing things come and go. By way of savasana, we experience death daily, and by its practice, embody the process of dissolution. Nothing is constant. Through *vipassana* (insight), we see that the world is actually showing us how to let go. Simple, poignant, but elusive, the Buddha taught, "All that arises ceases." Birth and death are a continuum. When we practice emptying before we begin, we are preparing to let go of whatever may come.

Emptiness lies at the very heart of the Great Teaching (Mahayana) of Buddhist practice. However, the term *emptiness* is mostly misconstrued, second only to the word *enlightenment*. People think emptiness is vacuity, blankness, nothingness, nil. In fact, emptiness is closer to receptivity. When we are empty, we are receptive, available, impartial, broad-minded, and tolerant. Paradoxically, emptiness is fullness. When we empty out, we feel full, spacious, open, and unconfined. When awakened in heart and mind, we feel fulfilled by each small thing—the shape of a cloud in the sky, the morning text from a sibling, a shared meal, a hug.

When we empty before we begin, we give back to the world. One of the oldest analogies for the mind in meditation is that of a mirror. When we discard our assumptions about things, we can reflect things as they are. If we only see the world through the narrow lens of "me, my, and mine" then we fail to live a full and boundless life. The American poet David Ignatow captured this so poignantly:

> I should be content
> to look at a mountain

for what it is

and not as a comment

on my life.[3]

As we brush the dust off the mirror of the mind (a classic analogy for clearing the junk, the "defilements" from the mind), we become more reflective. We can see the mountain for what it is: we bear witness to the heart pangs we feel in caring for an ailing mother ravished by dementia. We see the pain in our adolescent child, struggling to grow up in the world. We see the concrete sprawl of a the city overtake a fragile ecosystem.

It is difficult to realize the mirror-like nature of awareness. All too often we affix Post-it notes to the mirror of our mind. On those notes, we scribble down our jobs, our management strategies, our plans: pick up Jimmy from soccer; feed the dog; write thank-you note to Betty Sue; research online for a new vacuum; buy more Post-it notes. Over days, weeks, and months our notes pile up; they glom together like wet leaves until it is hard to see the mirror behind the notes. At times in meditation, we catch ourselves compiling a to-do list and we remove the note, but the adhesive backing leaves a sticky residue on the mirror. The habit of pasting our scribbles leaves a film (in yoga this mental residue is called *samskara*) so that in time we cannot see the clear, translucent, "empty" nature of mind.

By practicing yoga postures, controlled breathing (*prana-yama*), and heart-centered meditation (*metta*), we see through the tacky stuff of mind to the empty mirror. When I first began to practice meditation, I was always yearning to be free of thought, to be quiet and clear. This intention had merit because it prompted me to persevere and keep practicing. However, the yearning to be free of thought left a sticky imprint on the mirror of my mind. Each time I would come to the cushion I would desire to be silent and serene. Over time this craving left its mark so that each time I sat, I would get stuck on wanting to be free from being stuck! It is a common conundrum. It has taken me many years to let go of my gluey grasp and its sticky film on the mirror of my mind.

The experience of the mirror-like nature of the mind requires, at some point, a kind of surrender. The word *surrender* implies "giving over," as in the French word *render*, "to give back." For the first half of my spiritual journey, I never understood the significance of surrender. I thought it meant to give up, concede defeat, throw in the towel, and lose out. However, in the way that a mirror gives back whatever appears before it, surrender implies giving back that which does not belong to us. When we empty before we begin, we are ready, willing, and able to give of ourselves, to reflect back in kind.

There is another energetic quality we cultivate when we empty before we begin. Along with receptivity and surrender, we generate the spirit of forgiveness. On your morning cushion, it is helpful to embody the sentiment of forgiveness. This is not easy either, for in dark times when inhumane violence and cruelty are prevalent, it is difficult to forgive. In the still, quiet hours of my reflection, I take the word "for-giving" to mean "giving before." In meditation, I prepare to give to the world as much as my heart will allow on any given day. This is imperative on the path to building a Big Heart, a heart imbued with kindness, forbearance, resilience, and patience. If we do not kindle the fires of forgiveness, we are prone to moods, attitudes, and beliefs both cutting and negative. If we are not careful, we are quick to criticize and blame. When generating the spirit of forgiveness, we must first endeavor to forgive ourselves. We do this by accepting our own shortcomings, our own failures, our own mess. We for-give ourselves the space to be who we are. Each morning on the cushion we must breathe in forgiveness so that it penetrates down into our bones.

The Trappist monk Thomas Merton (1915–1968), a social activist, Zen practitioner, and man of faith, practiced inner communion. He sought the same space that yogis cherish for renewal, visions, and the simple joy of being. Through the practice of emptying, he entered what he called "the space of liberty," a heart-filled space yoked to the energy of love and possibility:

> The contemplative life must provide an area, a space of liberty, of silence, in which possibilities are allowed to surface and new choices—beyond routine choice—become manifest. It should create a new experience of time, not as stopgap, stillness . . . not a blank to be filled or an untouched space to be conquered and violated, but a space which can enjoy its own potentialities and hopes—

and its own presence to itself. One's own time. But not dominated by one's own ego and its demands. Hence open to others—*compassionate* time.[4]

Each morning we must enter this "space of liberty" for one half hour or more. We must set our devices aside and enter a wide-open landscape, full of potential. On this open ground we need not lay claim to anything. We enter a strange territory that has no authority, no ownership, and no rules. In Japanese Buddhism, this is the "pure land." In Vedanta, it is the *jivan mukti*—the space of self-liberation. All the twists and turns of the path, all the uphill and downhill slopes, lead to this space of liberty.

When I practice breathing, I focus on exhalation. If inhalation is the life-sustaining phase of the breath, exhalation is the letting-go phase. Exhalation is like an outgoing tide, ebbing away from the shoreline. Its movement draws us back to the ocean within. Dispelling the breath out of the body, is an act of letting go. For this reason, the exhalation can conjure fear and trepidation. It is always hard to let go of what we think we have and who we think we are, and this holds true for the breath. Only by exhaling can we truly learn to empty and be fulfilled by each passing thing.

In the morning, exhale repeatedly before beginning your day. In the evening, exhale before sleep, siphoning off the pressures that may have accumulated in your chest, abdomen, or neck. While driving to an appointment, exhale deeply before arriving. Exhale before moving into a yoga posture. At the very end of life, we exhale as we pass through the veil to the other side. The exhalation guides us back to the source from which we have come.

When I invite students to begin class in savasana I encourage them to drop their bones into the earth. I invite them to return to the "home" of their body, the "home" of their *prana* (life force). When the surging demands of the day overwhelm us, we must come back to the temple of our bones. We accomplish this by exhaling, emptying, and relinquishing the weight of our bones.

There is a well-known story in Indian mythology that speaks to this dissolution. Vishnu is the god who sustains the appearance of the world through the magic of his *maya*. Like an optical illusion, or special effect in a Hollywood blockbuster, the world is the work of his stagecraft, produced for a time and then made to vanish. Vishnu proclaims that at the end of time, everything returns to him.

> I am the cycle of the year, which generates everything and again dissolves it. I am the divine yogī, the cosmic juggler or magician, who works wonderful tricks of delusion . . . This display of the mirage of the phenomenal process of the universe is the work of my creative aspect; but at the same time I am the whirlpool, the destructive vortex, that sucks back whatever has been displayed.[5]

Each day we participate in the magical spin of creation. In time we see that reality is like a mirage, a concoction of the senses, a product of imagination. In the act of emptying, we let go of the delusion that sustains everything. This is why we practice savasana and learn to exhale. It is paradoxical to practice this pose at the beginning of a session. Yet there is tremendous power in letting go before you begin. Why wait until it is all over?

PRACTICE, INQUIRY, AND REFLECTION

IN MEDITATION

The Other Side of the Mountain

When you wake up in the morning, take your pee and go straight to your cushion. Don't make plans, don't check your mail or start sending and receiving. Don't look at the morning news. Stay offline. Choose a seat in an uncluttered part of your home, ideally away from books, appliances, and foot traffic. When you arrive at your seat, nestle in like a roosting hen. Settle into the weight of the bones of your feet, shins, and legs. Let your entire body come to rest. At the same time, lift your spine toward the sky. Imagine you are drawing a long and slender piece of grass upward from its sheath. Float the stem of your brain upward while casting your eyes downward. Look down into the center of your heart.

Sense the soft, steady breeze of your breath. With your lungs lifted and ribs wide, let your breath be delicate, steady, and light. Sense and feel the spaces between your ribs. Like a venetian blind whose horizontal slats open and close, open your ribs outward and upward as you inhale, and allow them to lower and contract as you exhale.

Relax your tongue, and release the short but powerful muscles that pin your mandible to your skull. Allow the skin covering your scalp to be supple, soft, and permeable. Empty all the air out of the sails of your lungs and exhale down to your nadir, down to the tip of your coccyx.

Rest in an uncluttered space of liberty by letting go of any agenda, strategy, or grand design. Sit in a spirit of receptivity, opening up to something just outside your control. Don't attempt to manipulate or micromanage your experience. You will only get in your own way and cause clutter. In the space of liberty, yoke to stillness, silence, and possibility. Spend time on the other side of the mountain, apart from the all-too-familiar terrain of "you." Empty before you begin, so that the flavor of openness stays with you throughout your day.

ON THE MAT

Savasana and the Art of Dropping

Lie in savasana with the back of your head supported by a blanket and a bolster tucked under your knees. Be sure you are warm enough; drape a blanket over yourself if necessary. As you lie down, allow your body to spread horizontally along the floor. Elongate the back of your legs by pushing out through your heels one at a time. Center your pelvis so that your sacrum spreads and widens against the floor. Lengthen the back of your neck by sliding your occiput (the bone at the back of your skull) away from your shoulders.

Savasana is the art of dropping. Allow the skin of your back to spread wide as it rests to the floor. Visualize the musculature of your legs releasing from your bones, like the flesh of a well-cooked salmon. Loosen your calf muscles, hamstrings, and gluteus muscles and permit them to give way and release to the floor. It is most important in savasana to relax the structures that surround the brain. Imagine the back of your skull to be like a ripe grapefruit, its rind leaving an imprint on the floor. Let the flesh of the fruit of your brain expand against the inside of your cranium. Let go of your jaw, tongue, throat, eyes, and inner ears. Become an empty vessel, spacious and bright.

Once you have reached a state of profound somatic quiescence, begin the process of letting go psychologically. This requires relinquishing your hold on things, people, and plans. Drop any attachment you have to material objects—your car, computer, kitchen, photo albums, and home. Know that when you die, you cannot take your laptop or smartphone with you to the other side! Then relinquish the ties you have to people, including friends and loved ones. Let go of the concepts, ideas, memories, and plans you may hold. Finally, discard any notion you have about spiritual accomplishment or revelation. Let go of who you think you are and who you think you ought to be.

OFF THE MAT

Engaged Letting Go

In the course of your day, practice engaged letting go. Prepare to give generously to each task, to everyone you meet, and to every passing circumstance. Engage fully with all your heart and mind. Put your passion into your living so that you are present for each passing thing. At the same time carry the spirit of letting go with you. Remember that each and every encounter is passing right before your eyes, like a bubble on a fast-moving stream. This does not suggest that you should be careless, irreverent, or detached. Practice right attachment, meaning give what you can and then let go. When I studied dance, one of my choreography instructors, Jonathan Wolken of Pilobolus, referred to this as "make it and break it." If you are overzealous and try too hard, you squeeze the moment and create tension. This is not good for you (as it can lead to great fatigue) or your partner. If you should let go too soon, you miss the moment and fumble your connection. Is your tendency to grip too hard, holding on to situations and people too long? Or do you tend to let go too soon?

This practice requires two opposing qualities—yielding and resiliency. By yielding you allow for spontaneity, expression, and connection. When yielding, you loosen the need to dominate, control, and lay claim to the moment at hand. Through resiliency you remain concentrated, present, and steadfast. This provides the determination and staying power to continue. Embody this spirit of yielding and resiliency in the marrow of your bones. Bone marrow is both solid and liquid. In the alchemy of the mind-body-spirit connection, your bones are the source of the deep life force, called the original *qi* in Chinese medicine. Resiliency is to be unwavering and solid, and yielding is to be fluid. Bring these qualities of solidity and fluidity to each passing thing as you practice engaged letting go.

2

Always New

WHEN WE WALK, we walk in the footsteps of our ancestors. Many have preceded us on the path, and the trail is well worn. We trust the way of the wisdom keepers who have worn the path step by step, for thousands of years. While we follow the way of those who have gone before us, our steps on the path are initiatory, always new. It is not that we are trying to replicate the walk of the Buddha, the guru, or the guide. In the yoga room, we are not trying to make a carbon copy of the posture that the teacher is demonstrating. On the mat today, our agenda is not to re-create the same posture we did yesterday. A wholehearted commitment to being on the path requires a willingness to tread in a way that is always and astonishingly new.

On the first half of the journey, we proceed like children, imitating what others have done before us. We may strive to execute a pose in precisely the same way that it has been shown to us. We copy the teacher, and we follow fellow students. I often see students in class copying the person in front of them, even if their fellow student is really out of position! There is nothing wrong with this kind of learning. At the start of the path, we all do this; we mimic our teacher in order to get the movement down. Without thinking, we do what we are told.

Inevitably, however, this brings up a big dose of self-doubt. *Am I doing it the way it should be done? Am I getting it right? Am I good enough? Are others doing it better than I am?* This kind of questioning can last for years. Some students never make it out of the mind-set of trying to do the movement correctly.

At the outset of our practice, we rely on the predictable, the routine, in order to become established. We conform to a particular pattern and repeat a set sequence. To make the practice stick at the beginning, we firmly adhere to the rituals, the book, the guide, the code, and the formulas. We "follow tradition," believing the method to be true. We get attached to our teachers and are loyal to their methods. While we generate conviction, we may have little tolerance for other traditions. In the beginning we rely on clear and solid boundaries, and we expect others to do the same. We form significant ties to our practice group and its purpose. We feel that we are "in," and we assume an identity within the "tribe," or *kula*. At the outset, our practice has the flavor of something very special. It may become a source of pride, self-assertion, even self-righteousness.

Later in our practice, we come to a crossroads where the exacting structure we have followed up to then must give way to a less formulaic approach. At this crossroads, we see that the first prescription for progress on the path may no longer serve us and that in fact the path to embodied wisdom requires another move, one that is less predictable and more elusive. What is necessary is a leap outside the familiar. While a flowchart that shows how to perform the movements is invaluable in the first half of the journey, it may not apply to the inner passage of the second half of the trek, which can be paradoxical and perplexing. On the path to embodying *prajna*, a Sanskrit word that roughly means "wisdom beyond knowing," the standards we relied on at first may no longer serve us.

The Middle Way teachings of the Buddha describe the trials of this very shift. Composed around the third century B.C.E. following Siddhartha's radical vision of the unity of all things, the Parable of the Raft is a delightful tale of two monks ferrying from the near shore to the far shore of a river. They carefully construct a raft both rigid and secure, one that enables them to make the arduous river crossing. The construction is elaborate and thorough, yet once they have traversed the body of water, the meticulously designed raft is to be abandoned. The story elucidates the teachings on nonclinging:

I have shown you how the Dhamma is similar to a raft, being for the purpose of crossing over, not for the purpose of grasping. Bhikkhus (monks), when you know the Dhamma (teaching, code of conduct) to be similar to a raft, you should abandon even the teachings, how much more so things contrary to the teachings.

If we are not careful, strict adherence to the raft leaves us standing on the far shore, urgently elevating the status of the raft, covering it in gold leaf, and safeguarding it at all costs. By clinging to the raft, we cannot travel on; thus our progress on the path is stunted. We may become defensive, dogmatic, and authoritarian. If we can integrate and include all that we have learned in the crossing without holding blindly to the devices that transport us, we open ourselves up to ongoing discovery and surprise.

In the journey onward, the real task is to make every moment new. That is, we must realize that it is impossible to replicate moments in time or to do things in the way they were done before. This applies to teaching. For instance, there are times when I think I have taught a really great class in my Tuesday morning time slot. The theme I used, the sequence I delivered, was just right. Then the following Tuesday I say to myself, "Ah, the class last week was great, so today I'll teach the same class just as before." Halfway through the class, I realize that I cannot repeat the experience from the week before. I instruct the same sequence and try to capture the same flow, the same spirit, but my class ends up feeling contrived, forced, and inauthentic.

You may know the expression "You can't step in the same river twice." The river of time is streaming past, and no two moments are ever the same. This is the very essence of the Tao. The Tao signifies the dynamic, creative, ever-changing nature of things such that all experience is likened to flowing water. Not only does the world around us change, but there is perpetual change inside our bodies. In this very moment, the spongy tissue of your lungs, the cells in your spleen, and the nerve fibers in your neocortex are in constant motion.

In this way, things are always new and happening for the first time. On the journey, we come to realize that every moment is fresh, spontaneous, and unconditioned. In our minds, however, we may assume that the experience we are having now is one we have had many times before. As a result, our lives appear boring, mundane, and monotonous. All too often, we find ourselves going through the motions. In any walk of life, this stifles the spirit and causes angst and suffering. When the spark of spontaneity is snuffed out, the essential life force wanes. The joy in authentic living is not to get stuck in the snare of habit but to find "always new."

There is an expression in yoga: *sadanava*. *Sada* means "ongoing, everlasting," and *nava* in Sanskrit shares the same origin as the English word "new." *Sadanava* suggests that things are constantly changing and eternally new. From the outer reaches of the galaxy to the blood vessels at the tip of your finger, nothing is fixed. To what extent we allow ourselves to be in the river of constant flux determines our overall quality of life. By living in the always new we feel more alive, more attentive, open to surprise and discovery. Yet how do we come to see the world as always new? This is why practice is important.

Everyone recognizes the reverberating sound of OM as integral to the yoga experience. The intonation of OM is one of the oldest and most widely practiced means of invoking the essential spirit of yoga. I think in every yoga studio from Tallahassee to Toronto, OM is called out at the start or end of a class. Why OM? What does it mean? This simple one-syllable mantra is called the *pranava*. *Nava*, as we have seen, means "new," and *pra* suggests "manifestation, coming forth, or being produced." The vocative OM is used to conjure creation itself. All manifestation—from the sound of the wind, to the cry of the newborn, to the clang of the recycling truck—is OM. The brush of the breath in the back of your throat on each inhalation and exhalation is OM. When intoning OM, all emanation throughout the universe is condensed into the vibratory power of a single sound. OM is charged with a creative power that gives birth to all things. By chanting OM, we are reminded that everything is perpetually happening anew.

In practice we learn to sense and feel that every breath, every pulsation, and every tremor across our skin is unique. It is as if we are leaves that have fallen onto a fast-moving stream. Suspended on the current, in the flow of the Tao, can I let go in the torrent of time? What if this very body and each and every breath is the actualization of time passing? There is an expression in Chinese Buddhism: "Make this very moment ten thousand years." In the perpetual flow of time, this very moment as you read is ten thousand years. The first morning light is ten thousand years. The breath you are on now is ten thousand years. We are part of a boundless flow of time.

A yoga posture is a perfect vehicle by which to observe the flow of the river of time. If I am in downward-facing dog pose (*adho mukha svanasana*), I listen to the current of my breath: sometimes rapid, sometimes shallow, sometimes still. I observe the expansion and contraction of my connective tissues. I sense the way that pressure continuously shifts as I bear weight in my shoulders. I observe the nuance of sensation that travels through my fascia, skin, organs, and joints. Different sensations arise as I stay in position for thirty seconds, one minute, two minutes, three minutes. Because the pose is constantly changing, it is always dynamic. To an outside observer, a three-minute pose may appear static. Nothing seems to be happening. Yet in the atmosphere of the inner pose, there is constant change. Like a meteorologist, I track the shifts in weather, including high and low pressures, humidity levels, wind variability, and temperature changes. In this sense, the atmosphere within me is shifting all the time. Without moving an inch, I travel miles and miles.

I am reminded of a video exhibit that I once saw at the Museum of Modern Art in San Francisco. The photographer had placed his camera on the Icelandic tundra over a twenty-four-hour period in late summer when there is perpetual light. Set in one spot, the camera captured the beauty of the enduring landscape: cloud cover came and went, shadows drifted, a glint of sunlight reflected onto a rocky bluff. There were subtle shifts in light between "dawn" (there was no night), midday, and 3 a.m. The video was displayed on the exhibit wall, which was the size of a roadside billboard. Shown in real time, the cycle for the entire "show" of the video footage took twenty-four hours. There were several comfortable couches in the exhibit, and so I sat and watched time slowly pass. It was a virtual meditation to witness the nuanced changes taking place in the natural world. I sat for forty-five minutes absorbed in a presence both vast and immense. A line from a Juan Ramón Jiménez poem entitled "Oceans" came to mind: "Nothing happens? Or has everything happened, / and are we standing now, quietly, in the new life?"

One of the primary ways to be on the cusp of change and to experience the always new is to decelerate, slow down, and bear witness to moments passing. Meditation requires an exquisite settling into stillness. When sitting on the cushion, I slow my respiration rate to that of a hibernating fish. Periodically, a big breath rolls through, and in its wake, my ribs, organs, and ligaments expand and resuscitate before settling down. I observe the way my thoughts meander like clouds, sometimes gathering into thick, ashen clusters and other times breaking into thin, wispy strands. As I drop further into the seated position, my heart rate slows, the peristaltic rhythms of my digestion become regular, and the neural firing in my brain goes silent. As time slows to a crawl, my awareness dilates. The aperture of my mind becomes far wider than my body, wider than place, date, and time.

When we do not slow down but rush headlong into our day, experiences get cemented together, like sedimentary rock—a mishmash of gravel, quartz, pebbles, and clay. It is hard to individuate one moment from the next, and nothing stands out clearly. When everything clusters together, held together by the glue of fear, anxiety, and pressure, we feel like we have no space (and no time) to witness anything anew. Somatically, experiences glom onto our jaw, neck, gut, and diaphragm making it hard to breathe. Under pressure the mind becomes muddled, calcified, and compounded. Without clarity of mind and space of heart, everything seems to stack up. Nothing we do makes us feel alive, and as a result, we feel disconnected, lost, and powerless. It is at these times that we need to pause. We need to return to the mat or cushion and proceed breath by breath and moment by moment in the flow of the ever-changing now. I often say that time, space and stillness are the greatest healers. The alchemy of time, space, and concentrated stillness can dissolve even the most lumpy, compacted states within the body-mind.

The always new is not simply an inspiring spiritual concept. It is actually the way things are. The Buddha achieved insight into the always new during his vision quest toward enlightenment, sitting from sunrise to midnight. He saw that all undergoes constant change, all is vanishing, and nothing is static. Every breath, every moment is vanishing and thus always new. In the wake of this insight follows the teaching of nonclinging. How can you cling when everything is in the process of change? Nonclinging, or nonattachment, lies right at the heart of all yoga practice.

Living the always new is to have an open state of mind without preconception. We call this beginner's mind. To have beginner's mind is to be receptive, sympathetic and open to ongoing change. It suggests being open to surprise. Marcel Proust, in his great work *Remembrance of Things Past* (also translated as *In Search of Lost*

Time), noted that the real voyage of discovery does not require visiting new landscapes, but in having new eyes. When the world is experienced through fresh eyes, everything appears vivid and bright. Moments we typically take for granted, like being on a bicycle, watching the flight of a bird, or breathing, become sources of subtle amazement.

In the midst of the daily round, it is common to get stranded in expectations about how things should be. It is then that we must realize that all things are a display of the always new. Like pressing the restart button on a computer, we return to beginner's mind. Meditation is helpful in this regard, for on the cushion we press the refresh button ten times, twenty times, or one hundred times. By returning again and again to the always new, we practice what many spiritual circles refer to as "being in the moment."

The aim of our practice is to always keep beginner's mind. This suggests a mind and heart that are open to possibility. Children experience the delight of the always new, readily feeling joy, loss, frustration, or pleasure. Adults typically classify and catalog experience into previously designated files. We box, fit, and label experience into categories in our minds. It is when we think we know how things are or how they should be that the spirited inquiry of the child wanes. I can recall a time in my childhood when I became convinced that in order to prove my worth, I needed to know the things of the world. I decided, somewhere in the wheelhouse of my eleven-year-old psyche, to become an adult and that meant leaving behind the playfulness and spontaneity of my child spirit. In substituting the supposed known for the mystery of the unknowable, I surrendered my beginner's mind. When we assume we know, we give up a world that is full of possibility. Thus practice involves relearning beginner's mind and being open to the always new. Called "original mind" in Zen, the spirit of beginner's mind invokes curiosity and wonder.

I think that a readiness and willingness to be surprised are necessary ingredients to leading a fulfilled life. But shaking off habitual tendencies is difficult. Neurologically, we get wired to respond today in the same way we responded yesterday. The circuitry of the brain gets programmed by "habit grooves" and defaults to connections that have been preestablished. I am sure you have heard the expression, "Nerves that fire together wire together," and thus the mind falls prey to the conditions that shape it. In this way, behavior becomes routine. In body-mind practices, we influence the flow of impulses through the connective tissues, nerves, glands, and viscera in order to generate new pathways. This steers us away from the "habit mind" and "habit body" toward an experience of the always new.

A yoga practice may become routine if we end up doing the same movements and the same kind of sequence over and over. Human beings are creatures of habit. In our exercise routines, we can become like gerbils in a cage, running in place on the spinning wheel. While it is good to have an everyday practice, there is a risk of going on autopilot. When a routine becomes repetitive, we move further away from intimate practice. Without listening and observing the changing weather patterns inside, a workout becomes another item we check off our to-do list. We simply go through the motions. It is then that we need to find new pathways of movement that illicit new sensations. There are myriad number of ways that nerves can wire together. A practice that aims to ride the changing edge is one that supports greater neuroplasticity in the nerves, fascia, and circulatory flow. This is important because how we practice determines how we live our lives. If our practice is mechanical, then our life becomes routine and wooden. In order to stay in the flow of the always new, in order to live life as an ongoing act of creation, it is critical to be on the cusp of constant change.

PRACTICE, INQUIRY, AND REFLECTION

IN MEDITATION

Beginner's Mind

Assume a comfortable position on your meditation cushion with your pelvis supported and your spine lifted. Become established on firm ground so that your bones settle into their support. Bring awareness to your breath so you sense each inhalation and exhalation as new. The beauty in breathing is that each breath is like a snowflake—no two are ever the same. Every breath is a new beginning, and with each breath we start over. Allow each breath to arise spontaneously out of the previous one.

Note how each moment, like every flake of falling snow, arises then dissolves. Directly experience a cascade of moments, recognizing that no two moments are the same. The Buddha's teaching, "all that arises ceases" suggests that each moment crystallizes as it comes into being, is here for a time and then vanishes. In the larger sense, reflect on the way in which everything is a unique pattern—one that takes form due to precise causes and conditions. Each delicate snow crystal moment has never arisen before and will never happen again. Note all the different patterns that appear while abiding in beginner's mind, free from interpretation and expectation. Avoid trying to make moments better, different, or more enlightened. Simply observe how moments arise then melt away. Become quite empty and available, not grasping or clinging.

If your thoughts pile up in zigzag patterns, then imagine your mind to be like the child's toy, the Etch A Sketch. The Etch A Sketch features two small knobs that can be turned to sketch lines and patterns onto the screen. When shaken, the screen returns to a clean, blank slate. Beginner's mind involves repeatedly going back to naught by emptying your screen and sitting without any obstruction in your mind. See the etches of your thoughts as mere patterns displayed on the screen of your mind. Beginner's mind is a very simple practice, but at the same time it is really advanced!

ON THE MAT

Be All Ears

Begin in child's pose (*balasana*). Set your knees hip-width apart and stretch your arms straight out in front of you on the floor, in the same way you stretch your arms in downward dog pose. Either support your forehead on the floor, or rest your head on a block or blanket. Enter the pose with beginner's mind—that is, "be all ears" and listen to the small, ongoing shifts that take place in your body. Note that every breath, every sensation is new. Scan your body for sensations and note whether your sensations are intense or mild. Observe where in your body you feel restriction. Explore the limitation or barrier within the stretch with a spirit of curiosity. Then note the places in your body where you feel ease and space. Where does it feel pleasant? Allow your awareness to absorb into the region of your body where you feel a positive sensory response. Ask yourself, *How does the interior of my pose change?* Note the feeling in your front hip crease, lower back, shoulders, arms, and hands.

Sense and feel any ongoing shifts within your breath, in the stretch of your fascia, the weight of your bones, and the contact of your skin. Be like a meteorologist, observing the changing "weather" in the pose; notice places of high pressure and low pressure. As blood infuses into your tissues, sense changes in the humidity levels of your body. Note any atmospheric changes in your neck and skull. Stay here for two minutes.

Now lie on your back in savasana with a blanket folded to a height of two inches tucked under your head. As you rest in stillness, note the pulses in your hands and wrists. Like a doctor of Ayurveda or Chinese medicine, take your own pulse by observing the pulses in your right and left wrists. Are your pulses more rapid or amplified on one side? Do they feel shallow, thin, wiry, flat, or thick? Note the way the back of your body drops into the floor. Imagine that your organs are like small water balloons, spreading as they release. Listen to the rise and fall of your breath and the weight of your ribs against the floor. What sensations can you feel in your chest? Sense the dance between your respiratory rhythm and your heart rate. Can you feel any pulses within your cranium? Visualize your brain suspended in fluid, held in place by sturdy ligamentous moorings. Sense the biodynamic pulse of your brain tissue as it continuously expands and narrows in response to the craniosacral rhythm.

Be like an ocean and sense the perpetual sway of circulating currents in your bloodstream, lymphatic channels, and nerve endings. Sense the fluid potency of all the cells and tissues of your body. Be all ears as you listen inwardly to the vital flow of prana through your blood and nerve channels (nadis)—circulating, evanescent, motile. Note the rise and fall of the waves of your breath. Absorb into the interior of your body that is always changing, always new. Stay here for five to ten minutes.

OFF THE MAT

At the Trailhead of the Eightfold Path

In the early Buddhist teachings, the path of the mind-heart is mapped with eight distinct routes. Each trail guides us from the ingrown, obsessive, myopic city of self into the raw power of the wilderness. On the trail we are not meant to fret about whether we have the right gear or ample food or worry about whether there are deadly snakes on the trail. This path is about being fearless in the open air, under the big sky. At the trailhead to the Eightfold Path, right at the get-go, the first trail posting is called Right View. Right View is perhaps better translated as Total View, or Big Vista—like a drone shot taken from above, you have to see the entire terrain. The first leg of the journey requires that you see all dharmas— all things—as impermanent, like drops of morning dew, flashes of lightning, or clouds. Each experience is like a cloud, gathering together and dispersing in time. You might recall cloud gazing and imagine seeing a seahorse, a gorilla, a young princess in the con- figuration of a cloud. The spectacle forms and within moments vanishes. In Total View, we come to see that everything is in the process of change. We realize too that everything is interconnected and that there is no such thing as a "me" separate from the ecology that surrounds me. In Total View we come to see everything anew.

As you set out on the path of your day, have the intention to live each instant with fresh eyes. This is the second trail posting of the Eightfold Path, Right Intention, or what I like to refer to as Yoked Intention. In your day have an altruistic motivation to be kind, to abandon negativity, and to practice nonclinging. Resolve to see every perception, thought, word, and deed as droplets of water, droplets of time, in the always new. In the Eightfold Path, each ensuing trail posting—Right Speech, Balanced Action, Right Livelihood, Balanced Effort, Total Mindfulness, and Yoked Con- centration—leads away from habitual, self-centered, and neurotic tendencies. Move slowly, listen with care, and have loving atten- tion. Be open to the always new and to the wondrous and strange grace of the world.

3

How Speed Gets
Trapped in the Body

WE ARE A culture of speed. The world today moves at such a
dizzying pace that it is difficult to avoid being pulled into a vortex
of speed. Thanks to the advent of the handheld "smart" phone, we
now carry implements loaded for high-speed connectivity everywhere we go—whether in large urban areas or rural towns we are
wired into high-speed grids. In this era of speed, we strive for con-
venience. We have groceries delivered to our door; we purchase
mobile tickets for faster trains that take us hundreds of miles in a
matter of hours; we use electronic personal assistants like Alexa,
Siri, and Google to access millions of facts in a mere few seconds;
we track weather systems halfway around the globe.

In Hindu cosmology, time is mapped out as a cycle of years, massive in number and scale. There are four ages, known as *yugas*, that depict the life cycle of the cosmos and the longevity of human civilization. The era we occupy now is called the Kali Yuga, the last of the four epochs of time. In the Kali Yuga it is said that the wisdom of the yoga teachings declines, widespread chaos and disorder prevail, and everything spins faster.

The culture of speed we occupy today is a recent phenomenon. Historically, human populations moved in time with the elemental world. Tribal people lived by the seasons, and their migratory movements were calibrated to the elliptical cycles of the planets. The body's delicate circadian clock—diurnal cycles of sleeping and waking—was set in accord with the varying light of the sun, moon, and stars. People had ample time to socialize, reflect, pray, and just be. They moved only as fast as the earth could spin.

In the accelerated pace of today's world, the body's physiological rhythms are amped up. Overwhelmed by speed, circulatory flow gets interrupted. Electrochemical signals, neurological firing, and the movement of fluids get thrown out of kilter. The *timing* involved in sleep, digestion, respiration, and hormonal balance gets thrown out of synch, compromising the body's capacity to self-correct or self-regulate. When caught in pressurized speed traps of stress and overwork, the body's homeostasis is disturbed. With speed trapped in the body, we are prone to sleeplessness, hypertension, inflammation, autoimmune disease, irritable bowel syndrome, chronic pain, and erratic temper. Aggravated by lifestyles of rush and under nearly constant pressure, cardiac arrest has become the leading cause of death in the Western world. Speed constricts the heart while amplifying pressure in the circulatory vessels throughout the body.

In keeping with the speed and velocity of the twenty-first century, it is no surprise that yoga classes today also move at a rapid-fire pace. It is the norm in power-flow classes for students to be moving almost constantly from the beginning of the class to the end. Caught in the vortex of speed, poses are done in a flash, and as a result there is little time to arrive, root downward, and be still. The primary objective of yoga, historically, has been to cultivate meditative awareness. This requires slowing down and waiting, watching, and listening to the vital rhythms that sustain us. In order to heal and rewire neuronal circuitry, it is essential to embody both physiological and psychological rest. When teaching yoga postures, B. K. S. Iyengar encouraged his students to find "the repose within the pose." As we hold poses longer, we cultivate the penetrating and imperturbable quiescence that is the hallmark of yoga practice.

Speed is antithetical to the practice of mindfulness. When we move swiftly, the world passes by in a blur. When we hasten through experiences, we fail to notice the nuanced expression of each passing thing. When we strive to get to our destination, the forward rush is all-consuming, and we only think about getting to where we are going. In the fast-track experience, we do not look around or take anything in. Caught in the trap of speed, we lose feeling and become anesthetized to the world around us. Speed inhibits contemplative awareness and stunts capacity for insight (vipassana). It is difficult to see clearly when we are moving lickety-split down the track.

When we move rapidly, it is also difficult to be conscientious. Under the sway of speed, we become desensitized to the environment. Whether in the use of natural resources, the consumption of food, urban development, or the building of sustainable relationships, we neglect to care for the world around us. When we move fast, we must inevitably watch out for ourselves. Speed tends to reinforce the importance of "me, my, and mine," for we become preoccupied with our own individual advancement.

Speed is addictive. When rushing becomes habitual, we hurry even when we have nowhere to go! Sometimes we go fast for no good reason. This is an example of how speed overwhelms the body; you may have had the experience of dashing to an appointment and getting stopped cold in traffic. You are anxious to continue your forward momentum, but all vehicles are gridlocked. While your car is standing still, inwardly your body continues to rev forward. Your breathing is rapid, your eyes dilate, and your heart rate amps up. This is an example of how speed gets trapped in the body.

We all have had this experience. Somatically it feels as if you are stepping on an accelerator while your engine remains idle. This phenomenon wreaks havoc on the body's internal systems. Like flooding a car's engine with gas, your body produces adrenaline, cortisol, and norepinephrine. Once this high-octane hormonal cocktail suffuses your bloodstream, it is difficult to shut it down or reverse its effects. Simply put, you get stuck in the "on" position.

Speed gets trapped in the diaphragm, fascia, gut, arteries, and nerves. Off the mat, when students of yoga hurry and rush, it causes the connective tissues of the body to seize up and tighten, limiting flexibility. When speed, intensity, and exhaustion build up in the body, layers of fascia bundle together, inhibiting metabolic flow. This causes tenderness and pain in the tissue and blocks the free flow of movement in a pose like downward dog as strain builds up in the shoulders, back, hamstrings, or feet.

In the onslaught of speed, it is hard to be present. This becomes all too evident in meditation. When we pause, sit still, and follow our breath, we feel overwhelmed by the traffic of our thoughts. Items on our to-do list, plans, past conversations, or money matters rush in, leading to restlessness, agitation, or pain. We may get pulled into a sinkhole of fatigue and feel sleepy and dull. Or we may crave to be somewhere else, anywhere other than where we are, inert and still. We feel frustrated at going nowhere. Sitting still we feel confounded at not getting ahead. As a result, we question the whole ordeal of meditation. How can the act of sitting idle have any value whatsoever? These reactions to slowing down are the classic "five hindrances" in the Buddhist teachings—craving, irritability, restlessness, listlessness, and doubt. Which of these five plagues you most?

When caught in the speed trap, the breath and brain are most susceptible to strain and dysfunction. Our lungs have an immediate and extensive connection to the outside air, and because lung tissue is highly sensitive, these organs are susceptible to distress. When speed gets trapped in the body, the delicate physiological rhythms that govern respiration get thrown out of synch. Under strain and duress, the diaphragm constricts, cinching in the ribs and chest cavity.

People inundated by speed are most vulnerable to a buildup of pressure in the head and are prone to what my Dzogchen teacher Tsoknyi Rinpoche called "brain squeeze." Intracranial pressure can lead to headaches, eyestrain, mandibular strain, and difficulty concentrating.

In physics it is well known that heat rises. When the body and mind are under stress, pressure and heat accumulate; like rising fumes, they invade the delicate structures of the cranium. One of the ways we restore cranial balance in yoga is to support the head with a prop. In postures like downward-facing dog pose or seated forward bend (*paschimottanasana*), a bolster or block placed under the forehead can pacify the connective tissues in and around the brain.

It is important to avoid rapid upward surges of movement into the head. In physio-spiritual practices like qigong and yoga, ascending "winds" are said to invade or "derange" the delicate brain circuitry.

In daily living, when friction accumulates due to speed, overwork, and tension, the delicate tissues of the brain are susceptible to irritation and constriction. Rapidly ascending "winds" are triggered by frustration, restlessness, and impatience. Internal surges of upward moving heat and pressure are carefully avoided in all the internal arts. In yoga, one of the "great seals," internal movements done to direct the flow of prana, involves moving the chin toward the sternum to prevent pressure from rising into the head (called net-bearer bond, or *jalandhara bandha*). There is a similar idea in Chinese medicine, where sudden upsurges of wind are known as "rebellious qi." Rebellious qi can lead to elevated blood pressure, migraines, and acid reflux. To counter this, all forms of qigong are designed to descend the life force into the lower belly, known as the *dantien*.

One of the primary aims of a regular self-care practice is to help reset the body's internal clock and support its regulatory functioning. This requires, first and foremost, slowing down. It is by slowing down that we return home and attune to the pulse of prana inside. When we slow down, we can practice the exquisite art of listening. In the hour of rush, it is most difficult to listen to the subtle flow of prana.

Rushing weakens our connection to the sublime, rarified force of the animating spirit. It was Thomas Merton who said, "Hurry ruins saints as well as artists. They want quick success, and they are in such haste to get it that they cannot take time to be true to themselves."[1] It is only by slowing down that we can hear the spirit whisperer inside. It is only in the depths of stillness that we detect the presence of something vast and subtle, something inexhaustible and immense, a pervasive force much greater than our own small self.

By slowing down, we penetrate through the multifold layers of self. These layers get pasted one atop the other like papier-mâché newspaper clippings plastered to the surface of a latex balloon. In slowing down we move through many lamina of text and image that come to define us. Our papier-mâché self is built up from layers of gossip columns, history records, current events, opinions, editorials, and advertisements. When we dare to go slowly, we begin to see the stories that define us. Through the yoga of insight, the outer coverings are loosened, while the glue that holds fast the pages of criticism and editorial reports cracks and chafes. Over time, the papier-mâché covering sloughs off so that the interior space of awareness is able to expand.

In meditation, when there is nowhere to go and nothing to do, we are forced to pay attention. One of the first things we may notice is how very difficult it is to pay attention. Caught in gusts of distracting winds, the "habit mind" scatters (called *citta vritti* in Patanjali's yoga). Accustomed to flitting from one thing to the other, the mind is unable to settle. Only by slowing down can we begin to yoke awareness. In the Eightfold Path of Buddhist training, this leads to what is known as *right concentration*. The contemplative travel writer Pico Iyer captured the critical link between slowing down, stillness, and concentration:

> In an age of speed . . . nothing could be more invigorating than going slow. In an age of distraction, nothing can feel more luxurious than paying attention. And in an age of constant movement, nothing is more urgent than sitting still.[2]

It is exhilarating to go slow. This is an oxymoron, the paradox of praxis. How do we feel invigorated by doing nothing? In China's fourth-century Tang dynasty, Taoist sages championed the art of doing nothing. In Taoism, nonstriving is paramount to practice. "If he acts without action (*wei wu wei*), then there is nothing that will not be in order," says the old book, the *Tao Te Ching*.[3] Only when we get out of our own way can tap the very source of all becoming. In being still and not exerting, we harness the essential potency known in Chinese medicine as the *original qi*. This spiritual potency cannot be cultivated when there is haste and overexertion. For those of us raised in the West, this is most difficult to fathom. We adhere to the notion that progress is made by bearing down hard, accelerating fast, and—NFL style—striving for the end zone.

Many moons may pass until you feel invigorated by going nowhere and doing nothing. Yoga is a time-honored practice, one that cannot be realized in a mere two hundred hours. Like fruit growing on the vine, a kind of ripening is required. Once the fruit has matured, it will drop of its own accord—without design, anticipation, or goal. We are all fruit hanging on the vine, and no matter how much we may insist, we cannot force the time of our release.

In my yoga therapy trainings, I like to say that time and space are the greatest healers. How do we allow time to do its good work? Rather than manage time, how do we allow time to work on us? Our lives often feel like a race against time. As we age, days spin by like fastballs. Days, seasons, and decades fly past. In the second half of life, we bear witness to the progression of generations: we shepherd our children to adulthood and minister to our dying parents at the end of their lives.

From time immemorial, yogis have known not to push the river of time, as it causes restlessness and haste and only impedes the migration of the soul. The art of practice requires "being in time," or better said, knowing that we are here only for the time being. In this age of speed, this headlong race into the future, we rarely live a day for the time being. We do not spend enough time simply being, without doing anything. Instead, we charge ahead at breakneck speed to keep up with the frenetic pace of the world. In this age of rush, nothing is more critical than moving slowly.

I must admit that slowing down is risky. It requires going against the prevailing high-speed connectivity of the time that we live in. There are occasions when I feel that if I relent and drop my pace, I will lose out and lag behind. This is a common angst of our time, that if we do not sustain our headlong rush, if we do not stay current, we will no longer be relevant. Pausing, slowing down, and being idle is antithetical to the high-speed pace of today's internet-mediated world. We become locked into systems that require us to "upgrade" every six months. Should we fail to upgrade our operating system, we no longer have access to the current information. If we don't upgrade, we essentially take ourselves out of the game. Inevitably this leads to feelings of loss, animosity, disenfranchisement, and isolation. It makes us feel "out of it."

As we race to keep up, I sense that we are all swept up in a whirlwind of collective grasping. Akin to a modern-day gold rush, we feel the urgency to stake our claim on the World Wide Web, promoting and profiting through Facebook, Instagram, Twitter, and Snapchat. Caught in a climate of heat and accelerated spin, we swirl like a tornado in a vortex of speed. In the wisdom teachings of yoga, this is called *samsara*. The word *samsara* has the connotation of revolving cyclically, going around and around without relief. When sucked into the spin cycle of samsara we suffer. We feel a sense of loss so acutely that we are prompted to go faster. The American psychologist and philosopher Rollo May wrote, "It is an old and ironic habit of human beings to run faster when we have lost our way."[4] Why do we do this? What prompts the impulse to accelerate when we are under threat? Perhaps it's that we cling to that which is fleeting. We cling to our bodies, our possessions, wealth, notoriety, beauty, and success.

The culture of speed now threatens the very equilibrium of the planet. Collectively we must slow down so we do not burn ourselves up. We must slow our consumption of natural resources. We must slow the rate and volume of carbon emitted into the atmosphere. This is an enormous task, but it is our calling to carry it out. There are numerous ways to participate in this slowdown, including the slow food and slow building movements. How do we take our foot off the accelerator? It begins in the body by slowing the heart rate, reducing the sympathetic drive (responsible for the flight-or-fight response), slowing the breath, lowering blood pressure, and sleeping longer and deeper. On the mat, we learn to break out of the "habit body" that is compelled by urgency and motivated by acquisition. We must learn the art of being through ease, stillness, and silence. In yoga this is called *satchitananda*— the joy of just being. I sense that a downshift is possible when I use a meditation app to track how many other people worldwide are sitting. When the meditation tracker vouches that there are 416,000 people sitting at the same time, I feel a surge of optimism that it might be possible to decelerate and, in so doing, collectively wean ourselves from the speed habit.

PRACTICE, INQUIRY, AND REFLECTION

IN MEDITATION

Slowing the Rush—A Deceleration Asana

Begin in any seated position that is stable and comfortable. Align your cranium over your torso and your torso over your pelvis. In the first three or four minutes, take time to settle into the weight of your legs. Sense the weight of your legs settling downward to the floor. It is said in the *Tao Te Ching* that the root of lightness is heaviness. Visualize your legs underground, as if you are subterranean from your navel downward.

When speed gets trapped in the soft tissues, it typically causes cervical strain and cranial compression. Release any clenching in your mandible, throat, tongue, cranial bones, and upper neck. Release all the skin around your ears and allow the portal of your inner ears to soften and widen. When speed gets trapped in the diaphragm, it inhibits the natural flow of breath. Pay attention to the soft, light flow of your breath. Sense the elasticity of your diaphragm at its outermost edges where it inserts into the margin of your internal ribs. This is the most mobile part of your diaphragm and its motion will allow your breath to become long, fine, and subtle.

Then visualize your skull and upper torso to be the shape of an hourglass, a tool that has been used since antiquity to mark the passage of time. Visualize the upper sphere of the hourglass at your head, the narrow middle at your neck, and the lower sphere in the region of your chest. In your mind's eye, turn the hourglass upside down so that, grain by grain, the sand trickles out of the upper sphere of your head through your neck and into the lower sphere of your chest. As the grains of sand drop from your head into your chest, generate a feeling of fullness in your heart. As you slow the rhythm of your breath, mark the slow descent of time moment by moment, grain by grain. Let all thoughts, memories, and concepts siphon out of your cranium. With each passing grain, permit a quality of deep rest to penetrate the skin of your face, scalp, sensory organs, and brain tissue.

As you invert the hourglass, visualize your skull becoming transparent, like the empty space of the upper sphere of the glass. The bones of the skull are delicate and exquisitely crafted to accommodate slight changes of pressure within the cranial orb. All too often, when speed gets trapped in the body, the cranial bones constrict. This compromises the motility of the brain tissue, that is, its capacity to expand and contract naturally. Sense the way the bones on the sides of your skull widen—the temporal, parietal, and sphenoid bones. Generate a feeling of lightness and spaciousness within these bones and at the opening to your ear. The temporal bones are the primary bones in the body that signify the progression of time. As the hourglass of your skull empties, experience timelessness and space. Sense a luminous, translucent quality to your awareness. Rest in the spaciousness of a deep, abiding stillness.

ON THE MAT

Bridge to Light and Space

In this practice, be sure you warm up with several gentle back arches, including lunges, warrior I pose (*virabhadrasana* I) and cobra pose (*bhujangasana*). Then prepare for supported bridge pose (*setu bandha sarvangasana*). Place a bolster or set of folded blankets six to ten inches thick under your pelvis as you recline. If you do not have a bolster, place a yoga block under your sacrum; however, the bolster is softer and less likely to cause strain. Be sure the prop is positioned in the center of the back of your pelvis. Lie back with your shoulders on the floor and the back of your head resting on the mat. Remain with your knees bent for several minutes drawing your breath into your chest and abdomen. Slow your breath so it is long, fine, and subtle. Bridge pose creates both vertical extension and lateral spreading through the torso. In the back arch, the region of the kidneys and adrenal glands passively contracts. This helps to regulate adrenal function. At the same time, generate a feeling of ease and suppleness in your throat as it softly squeezes closed (this is a preparatory movement for jalandhara bandha). This impacts the thyroid gland that is chiefly responsible for metabolic flow in the body. When speed gets trapped in the body, the adrenal-thyroid loop is often disrupted, resulting in low energy and fatigue.

Stay in this pose for several minutes. Then extend your legs by pushing out through your heels while drawing your toes back toward your head. Avoid back pain by actively stretching the backs of your legs. Be sure your legs are slightly wider than hip-width apart. This introduces a lateral expansion in your lower abdomen, spreading wide the region of the powerful iliopsoas muscle and endopelvic fascia (surrounding the uterus, bladder, and colon). Breathe slowly, expanding your upper abdomen and chest cavity.

This pose helps to dissipate any strain that may have accumulated in your gut, diaphragm, or cardiovascular system. Cultivate space in your abdomen and chest while remaining completely passive in your neck and skull. After remaining with straight legs for several minutes, bend your knees and slide the bolster out from under you. Then come up to sitting. Note the way your entire trunk feels light and spacious.

OFF THE MAT

When Caught in the Vortex of Speed

As you travel through your day, notice the frequency in which you get caught in vortexes of speed. You may find yourself in traffic, hustling late to an appointment, or hastily shooting off last-minute messages. Notice what happens to you somatically when you are pressured by time and scrambling to get things done; feel the epinephrine speeding through your blood. What happens in your body when you feel such urgency? How does it impact your gut, neck, and eyes? When speed gets trapped in the body, it often lodges in the soft tissues just above and below the diaphragm. Above the diaphragm, stress increases the rate and force of contraction of the heart. Below the diaphragm, speed causes constriction in the vulnerable tissues of the solar plexus.

Notice how rushing separates you from your body. What changes occur in your respiration, blood pressure, and skin temperature? Each of us has a neurological center that acts as a magnet for stress. Note whether one of your chakras—your brain, eyes, throat, heart, or belly—habitually holds stress. When caught in a speed vortex, do you accelerate more? Does your mind become blurry like the static on a television screen? Or when overwhelmed, do you become airborne and lose touch with your immediate environment? In the clutch of unrelenting urgency, it may be hard to feel anything. Track your somatic experience inside the speed vortex as best as you can. Slow down your experience by bringing awareness to your breath, heart rate, and blood pressure. Teach yourself to deescalate by shepherding your awareness back to the present moment. Decelerate your experience by feeling your feet on the floor, noting the rise and fall of your breath, and visually registering detail in your immediate environment. This will help siphon strain out of your body and bring you back to present-moment awareness.

4

Right Effort

IN THE FIRST half of my yoga journey, I was drawn to a high-octane, power practice. I was fervent about making progress and was on a trajectory of upward mobility through the order of poses. It was the kind of practice where students looked like they were in gym class—donning sweatbands, carrying towels, and wearing skimpy clothes. I was fervent, disciplined, and competitive. Inwardly I competed against myself, eager to better myself. Outwardly I would compare myself to other students on the mat. The practice was a rite of passage, testing myself through strenuous and acrobatic poses. I was eager to prove myself and receive validation from the guru and fellow students alike. The more strength and flexibility I mustered, the more I advanced through the system. I grew attached to the system, felt loyal to its methodology, and ardently defended the techniques and protocol we used in practice. I felt that I had found my tribe. Inspired by the mantra, the specialized breath work, and the flow of poses, I took on the identity of the tribe. I wore Indian clothing, became a strict vegetarian, and learned Sanskrit.

In these beginning years, multiple hidden forces were at work within me. Had I been striving since grade school in this same way? What ghosts within my personal history was I exorcising? I felt compelled to pass through a ring of fire and burn my old identity in favor of a new, more spiritually appealing one. All the while, I was operating from the willful urge of my own striver.

This chapter explores the critical ways that we must work with our inner striver to find right effort. This is challenging, as the demands and pressures to succeed in today's world necessitate a well-honed striver. In order to pay for a mortgage, cover health insurance, eat well, and have enough financial reserves to vacation once a year, we must apply ourselves rigorously. From third grade on we learn to strive for the gold star in class, to pirouette perfectly in ballet class, and to boot the kickball as far as we can on the playground. So it is not a surprise that beginning students of a transformational path like yoga set out to achieve and "master" the poses.

The will to perform and make progress has a long and enduring history in America. When Europeans first arrived on the American continent, pilgrim communities advocated dutiful and strenuous work, hard labor, and, above all, "good works." This was a motivating ethic: the more diligent and hardworking people were, the more likely they were to align their moral compass to God's will and achieve salvation. They thought they could influence their own personal destiny, their karma, via hard work: since God worked through them, the Puritans were exercising God's will. This belief is still rampant today, as people strive to build their stock market portfolios, buy bigger houses, and gain a step up the social ladder.

However the quest to realize the state of yoga necessitates something altogether different. While some effort is certainly required, one cannot simply apply a Calvinist value system to a yoga practice and expect to achieve enlightenment. For those of us raised under the influence of the Protestant work ethic or in a Judeo-Christian background, there is an implicit motivating drive to succeed. This drive has tremendous sway over much of the population, motivating people's thoughts, beliefs, dreams, and goals. In a culture of strivers, success or failure, gain or loss, good or bad are always on the line. The pervasive influence of this force goes largely unacknowledged until, in quiet moments of reflection and contemplation, you shine the lantern of your awareness on your own inner striver.

In the second half of my practice life, I have spent precious time reflecting on the origins of my own inner striver. My father was an ordained minister in the Presbyterian Church, as was my grandfather and his father before him. Even though I was not actively raised in a church community, the Protestant ethic circulated through my bloodstream. When I first began yoga, invisible forces urged me on, motivating me into handstands and backbends. I was under the spell of familial and cultural assumptions as I strived toward gain and sought approval. These were forces that had been set in motion long ago, persuasive forces much bigger and more impactful than my short lifetime.

It has taken me many years to be able to identify the underlying forces at work in me. This reckoning has required patience, perseverance, and real faith. Countless times I have posed these questions to myself: *What am I yoking to? Who is the striver? And what is there to gain?* It has been like an archeological dig, sifting through layers and layers of personal history. In the way that an archeologist excavates an ancient site using small picks, trowels and brushes, quarrying the depth psyche requires painstaking and delicate work. Through contemplation and insight meditation, I have sifted through many layers of karma—hope, fear, and longing that left their imprints on the soft sand of my soul.

I think each of us is replete with artifacts from our familial and cultural ancestry, encoded like DNA into our skin, bones, and flesh. When we first adopt Eastern practices, such as yoga or qigong, we attempt to break free from the archival material of our personal history. While the first half of a practice may involve assuming the garb, speaking the lingo, and performing the exotic rituals of a foreign land, in the second half of the journey we must circle back home to integrate the personal history of our own signature self.

The practice presents an opportunity to wrestle with our angels and demons and work through the hidden forces that have had dominion over us. Yet in no way will sheer force provide the kind of breakthrough that yoga requires. For ultimately, any attempt at self-mastery and any practice designed to enhance one's personal power, assumes the ego's own likeness. The soul-self, on the other hand, does not bloom by the will's volition. Something outside the scope of our own doing, and always just beyond the grasp of the ego, is required.

If they are not careful, pushers get increasingly better at pushing, and as a result they know no other way of practicing. This is hard to reconcile, for more often than not, compulsive effort is a source of approval and reward such that pushing becomes self-perpetuating. Bewitched by their own power, achievers are typically reluctant to relinquish their purposeful, driven approach. Yet only by recalibrating the very impulse that feeds their prowess and self-worth can they begin the profound work that involves risk, trust, loss, and humility.

The challenge of working with the striver is not merely a twenty-first-century dilemma. On the map of the Eightfold Path, right effort speaks to the importance of not pushing too hard, on the one hand, and not conceding to sloth and torpor, on the other. The Buddha knew all too well the pitfalls of excessive effort. At the outset of his spiritual quest, he put himself through trials of extreme severity and self-punishment. He attempted to overcome his body and mind by force of will through *tapas* (asceticism). Through fasting, pranayama, and yoga, he pushed himself to the brink of self-immolation. Having suffered and endured corrosive self-mortifying practices, he later espoused the Middle Way, which favors neither indulgence in sense pleasures nor strenuous, backbreaking practice.

In the course of a day, whether on or off the mat, right effort requires moment-by-moment negotiation. We must ask ourselves, *Am I overexerting? Or am I too passive?* Right effort (or what I like to think of as balanced effort) is not a practice that we realize once and for all and then move on. We must embody balanced effort in the way we exercise, study, raise our children, communicate with our employer, and wash the dishes. In yoga, we must seek the middle ground of right effort within every pose, every pranayama breath, and in every attempt to quiet the flurry of thought in meditation.

In the way that an archer strings a bow, right effort requires careful listening to the pressure, tension, and torque within a pose. Over time we learn to string the bow with just the right amount of force so the stretch has "right tension." If there is too much effort, the pose becomes rigid, clenched, and aggressive. If there is too little effort, the pose becomes lax and inattentive. The art of practice is to learn precisely where to engage and where to release. For example, if I am in shoulderstand (*sarvangasana*), it is critical that I keep my throat, eyes, and face soft. I release any grip in my chest, diaphragm, and internal organs. However, I actively engage my inner legs and powerfully lift my tailbone. Thus right effort requires simultaneously engaging and letting go. It necessitates attentive listening to the small shifts that occur in the respiratory rhythm, the stretch of fascia, and the pressures within the joint capsules. Right effort requires continuous internal adjustments to insure the free flow of prana in the blood, lymph, and nerves.

Realizing right effort in the arc of daily life is critical to well-being. Off the mat, when we push too hard, we are prone to stress, anxiety, and exhaustion. On the other hand, when we fall short and fail to apply ourselves, we may never realize our potential. Skillful action suggests the delicate balance between alertness and ease, resiliency and yielding. Right effort must be fueled by enthusiasm, focus, endurance, and grace.

One of my teachers described right effort as a combination of tension and laxity, or "tight-loose." This suggests both readiness and relaxation. When we discover the very fine balance between effort and ease, resistance and receptivity, control and surrender, knowing and not knowing, we embody the Middle Way. This exquisite balance lies right at the heart of yoga practice.

Before arriving in the middle, I spent many years experimenting with extremes. Not only did I practice extreme poses (and survived), but I was also extreme with my diet, rigid in discipline, and strict in my ideals and judgments. At times I would project my narrative of idealism outward onto others, yet more often than not, my extremism was inwardly directed. Eager to make progress on the path, spiritual aspirants, or what Robert Bly called "spiritual ascenders," are often inwardly demanding. If not careful, inward pressure can give way to self-punishing thoughts, attitudes, and behaviors. Living under the weight of internal expectations, real or imagined, we are prone to harm ourselves. Thus the Buddha's directive to live the Middle Way was meant to steer practitioners away from severe attitudes of self-condemnation, self-denial, and self-abuse.

It must be said that effort is a critical ingredient to yoga practice. In the ritual origins of yoga, tapas was necessary to effect change. In ritual alchemy, tapas is heat and combustion and enables transubstantiation from one chemical state to the next. Without tapas, there is no change. Tapas can occur on both physical and psychological levels. For instance, in the body, tapas occurs at the cellular level as the molecule ATP is converted to energy and as ingested food is converted to blood in the intestines. On the psychological level, tapas is required to turn anxiety, obsession, fear, or self-condemnation into a more open, uninhibited state of mind. In yoga, tapas is zeal, ardor, and fierceness. It is Siva in the ring of fire, dancing his ritual dance of creation and destruction.

At some point in the course of a prolonged yoga practice, each of us must enter the ring of fire. We burn through physical impurities and the overgrowth of mental fixation. Sometimes, unexpectedly, the world singes us, as when we receive a frightening physical diagnosis, our marriage breaks down, or we experience the loss of a loved one. But yogis routinely go straight into the ring of fire to change themselves.

Along with tapas, the effort required to effect change in yoga is called *virya*. Virya is zest, fortitude, and potency. It is the brawn of the warrior in warrior pose and the muster required for the handstand (*adho mukha vrksasana*). In the beginning of a practice, we build virya in the postures, gaining the confidence and strength required to move through states of blocked physical tension. In the latter half of the journey, we develop psychic virya through introspection, that is, we open the eye of wisdom to see through the obscurations that cast a shade over our hearts and minds. Spiritual virya is necessary to move from self-serving small-mindedness to kindness and empathy.

When the scales of balanced effort tip toward immobility, the spark of virya must be ignited. All the yoga texts warn us about the dangers of lethargy and doubt. These are two of the five classic hindrances on the path to awakening. Dullness, complacency, and depression stifle the spirit and leave us feeling disempowered. Today despair, fatigue, and depression plague the old and young alike. When confined to the dark (called *tamas* in Ayurvedic psychology), the prana is dampened, and attempts to rekindle the flame of ardor and passion can feel like an overwhelming task. Torpor flattens prana. Thus we do practices to stretch and strengthen the connective tissues in order to amplify the prana inside. An emboldening teacher, an inspiring sequence of poses, or a heartening meditation can help energize (or "pranagize") the animating spirit within.

It may be that the fire in the heart has been snuffed out. All too often this happens in childhood when a child's spark of exuberance and passion is extinguished by an overly controlling parent, coach, or sibling. Sometimes self-expression is stifled by an authoritarian and dogmatic religious institution. Trauma can squelch the raw, native potency of a child, a potency that includes endurance, vitality, and courage. When beginning a practice that involves physical, psychic, and emotional transformation, it may be necessary to do repair work first in order to revive the source of vitality within. When the body-mind has been frozen and immobilized, right effort is necessary to revitalize and heal.

Across many styles of practice today, power is associated with yoga. Both men and women are drawn to power yoga as power legitimizes, emboldens, and provides a means to self-possession. Power practice can provide students with the necessary determination and fortitude to begin to heal their divided self. Yet some never make it beyond the identity of power that is produced from the early years of practice. It is tempting to adhere to the seeming authority that power gives us. Power has allure and magnetism and can elevate us in ways previously unimagined.

Akin to the challenge of actualizing right effort, realizing "right power" is elusive. This is partly due to the fact that as a culture, we are geared to power. We are goal-oriented; we value achievement, pursue rewards, and make the long climb up the ladder of success (if the ladder is available to climb—not all communities have access to the ladder). Power is seductive. Both personally and collectively we are drawn to it. Yet how does the quest for power fit into the cultivation of yoga? Does it augment progress on the path or does it detract from self-realization?

In the second half of the journey, physical virya becomes far less significant. Ironically, we come to a point where we are willing to abdicate the very same power that has served us for years in practice. We move from outer strength to inner humility, realizing that ultimately, our individual power is limited. Often it is a break, an injury, a loss or failure that forces us to see the limitations of our own small self. This is often a painful, if not bewildering, turn in the road and is one that most of us avoid as best we can.

As we have seen, our attempts to achieve may either fortify

the ego or deflate it. Many of us get entangled in the net of self-worth, which is contingent upon our capacity to perform in the world. This is inherently problematic when it comes to the domain of spirit. For spirit cannot be captured by sheer force of will in the way a rodeo rider ropes a bull. It cannot be accomplished, owned, or occupied. This is a challenge, for the prerogative of the ego is to rope in experience, to colonize whatever it may encounter and identify it as "me, my, or mine." When the ego pursues the goal of yoga, it inevitably leaves its own mark, its own imprint. Instead of meeting spirit face to face, the ego simply encounters some version of its own likeness. The very effort to attain the state of yoga, and the seeking itself, obscure the path to realization.

Self-inquiry and reflection are essential on the path of yoga, and right effort plays a vital role in these practices. While effort in meditation is necessary (effort is required to land your buttocks on the cushion for half an hour each day), real finesse is required to yoke mindfully without grasping. On the meditation cushion, right effort is somewhere between focusing hard to concentrate the mind and spacing out altogether. We spend hours on either side of this divide until we land spontaneously, without thinking, smack-dab in the middle.

This is the crux of yoga training: to see the indivisibility of all things without getting blindsided by our own small point of view. At some point on the path, we must cross over the divider that seemingly stands between us and the rest of the world "out there." On the path of yoga, we all must pass through this gate en route to the experience of the unified, boundless self. There are innumerable techniques and instructions for how to make this crossing: meditation, Zen koans, chanting the name of God, holding your breath, reciting a mantra, visualization, nondual awareness, and so on.

In the second half of our journey, it is most queer and extraordinary that when opening to mystery and the strange way of grace, not-doing is equally as important as doing. In the same way, inaction is just as important as action and not-getting is as essential as getting.

In the Taoist practices of China, noneffort is celebrated as essential to embodiment of the Way. It suggests following the natural course of things, in the way that water yields to river stones, the breath moves in and out, and blood flows in our bones. The Tao flows of its own accord. Any attempt at controlling or manipulating the fundamental essence presents an obstacle to its path.

At some point we come to realize that the fundamental animating force of the universe is much bigger than we are, and any attempts to locate or grasp it are futile. In order to directly experience the raw, empty, immeasurable force that is the origin and dissolution of all things, we are best served by getting out of our own way. It is by not-doing and nongrasping that the magnificent force of the universe (*mahashakti*) flows through us.

For years I found nondoing to be a strange and perplexing practice. At the outset of my journey, I assumed that progress is always made by getting further. Why would spiritual training be any different? Habituated to the use of effort, I thought nondoing to be a waste of time. I had no way to relate to not-doing, for I had invested years in achievement through command. It has taken me a long time to come to appreciate not-doing and to realize the merit of not trying to achieve anything. Contrary to all my assumptions about how to make headway on the path, I have found that not-doing enables access to a whole new dimension. Critically, it gives access to the other side of the mountain, just beyond the reach of the scheming, planning, volitional ego. I came to realize that any attempt I might muster to engineer the state of enlightenment was doomed.

Through right effort, we come to a part of the journey that the ego-self could never imagine. We enter territory where there is nothing to get or grasp, and there is no more becoming. With the mind empty and attentive, we come into a presence that evades definition and cannot be put into words. It is a strange state of grace, one that always escapes definition. It is like being filled by vast, wondrous, open space.

PRACTICE, INQUIRY, AND REFLECTION

IN MEDITATION

Not Too Tight, Not Too Slack

Begin by sitting comfortably on a support so that your spine is upright. In the first minute, be sure that your sitting bones ground evenly and that you lift upward from your lower back. Start by relaxing your tongue and jaw as stress and strain often accumulate in the mandible. Yoke your attention very lightly to the rise and fall of your breath. In the first five minutes, actively concentrate your awareness. You might count your breath up to five, such that each inhalation and exhalation together make one cycle. When you reach the count of five, begin the count again. With each ensuing breath, see that your attention becomes lighter, finer, and clearer. Once you have achieved a steady state of awareness, discontinue the process of counting and rest in open awareness. Practice right effort, avoiding mind traps—sinkholes and ditches—that pull you down and cause you to be inattentive.

As you settle, let go of any attempt to improve or further yourself. Gradually reduce any effort to become better, more advanced, or enlightened. Rest in clear and spacious awareness. Avoid trying to get anywhere or become anything. Watch carefully, for the mind is obstinate and persuasive, and it will dupe you into trying to achieve the goal. The side of you that is used to making progress will feel confounded. Your inner striver will not know what to do. Be super patient and super still. Let go of all efforts toward gain or fulfillment.

At the same time, effort is required to prevent your mind from wandering. It is like fishing. If you hold the fishing line too tightly, it will appear unnatural to the fish and you will never catch one. If your hold is too slack, you will never feel the fish at the end of your line. Find the delicate balance between holding your attention too tight or too slack. Know that at times your attention will likely be too taut and your effort excessive. Build confidence in the fact that if you micromanage each moment and strive too hard toward the goal, there is no way you will find it. However, take care not to become distracted, too relaxed and dull. In each moment, find the middle ground of right effort.

Stay here for twenty to thirty minutes, and then rest at the end in savasana.

ON THE MAT

Pranayama

Begin pranayama practice by lying on a bolster or folded blankets elevated four to six inches off the floor, so that your entire spine is supported. Place a small blanket or towel under the back of your head so that your cranium is propped upward and slightly higher than your neck. Be sure that your spine is centered on the bolster and that your lungs spread laterally away from the midline. Widen your lungs like the broad, green leaves of a banana tree.

Once you lie down, allow your body to be completely still and observe the fluid movement of your breath. At the start, breathe naturally, letting your breath flow of its own accord. Sense and feel the texture and consistency of your breath as it brushes against the back of your throat. Remain for several minutes simply observing the inherent motion of your breath.

Then bring your awareness to your inhalation. Observe the beginning, the middle, and the top of your in-breath. Carefully, and with real finesse, actively expand your inhalation. In the same way that a balloon fills with air, sense the expansion of your lungs against your back ribs, side ribs, and front ribs. Practice right effort as you breathe in. Avoid being greedy and forceful by attempting to take in the maximum amount of air. This violates the spirit of pranayama. Rather, yield to the breath in the way that tall grass yields to the wind, moving in time with the current of the air. Right effort requires exquisite listening. If you overexert in pranayama, it will cause strain in your intercostal muscles, your diaphragm, and the visceral membranes around your lungs and heart. Use just the right amount of force to expand. Pranayama should never be conducted through willful effort.

Now breathe in halfway, pause, and retain your breath for several seconds. Breathe in again toward the top of your lungs. In the pause, allow your awareness to soak inward. The more you are able to soak inward, the more you will relinquish control over your breath.

Next divide your inhalation into two parts, pausing first at 30 percent capacity, then again at about 60 percent capacity, before breathing to the top of your lungs. Have an intention to *receive* your breath rather than striving to fill your lungs to capacity. Find right effort in pranayama, the delicate middle ground between too much effort and too little. Practice this technique for ten minutes before letting your breath return to normal. Lie in savasana for several minutes before coming up to sitting.

OFF THE MAT

Right Tension

This practice involves manifesting right effort in the flow of your daily life by bringing awareness to the occasions when you either try too hard or are too passive. In any situation—whether at work, in conversation, in a meeting, or when driving—note the occasions when you apply too much force. Often this is accompanied by feelings of urgency, impulsiveness, and impatience. Note that when you put undue pressure on yourself or others, an underlying attitude of craving or grasping is involved. What happens in your body when you try too hard? Do you notice constriction in your gut, eyes, or jaw? Does heat accumulate in your body? Are you compelled to push too hard at certain times and with certain people? That is, do recurring circumstances trigger the pusher in you? Note that the strong energy of exertion is seductive, and once instigated, it is difficult to relent. Overexertion leads to fatigue in the body and mind. Become aware of the moments in your day when you feel both "wired and tired."

Conversely note the times in your day when you do not make enough effort to be present. You might space out and avoid a person or situation. You might become distracted and absentminded. When you exhibit a lack of effort and lose connection to yourself and others, note the way you feel inside. Do you feel lost, detached, or isolated? If your concentration wanes and you lose attention, what happens in your body? Do you feel spacey, distracted, withdrawn, or restless?

Right effort is critical for the practice of present awareness. In the midst of changing circumstances, right effort demands moment-by-moment negotiation of your physical, emotional, and mental vitality. As you respond to situations that arise, is it your propensity to overreact or to underreact? In the flow of your daily life, right effort suggests interfacing with the world with just the right amount of tension. In the practice of right tension, embody a relaxed concentration, neither too slack nor too taut.

5

The Quest for the Perfect Pose

THOSE WHO BECOME deeply committed to yoga and devote hours and hours on the mat—refining their breath, balancing on one leg, and working to make their minds still—are often motivated by strong tendencies toward perfection. The desire to purge mental and physical impurities holds real allure. Students strive to become healthy and beautiful and master of their bodies. Longing for an uncorrupted state, free from contamination, students attempt to live up to a grand ideal, wherein the body, mind, and emotions are composed and equanimous. Inwardly they seek solace; outwardly they wish for a world order that is balanced and harmonious.

When the yogic teachings collide with the urge to be pure,

faultless, and true, it is a veritable perfect storm. All too often, a yearning for purity, ingrained somewhere in the depths of our psyche, finds an outlet in yoga techniques—techniques that espouse cleanliness, equilibrium, and peace. For those raised in middle- to upper-class backgrounds (by far the majority of the population filling yoga classes, retreats, and festivals today), there is a longing to be virtuous and desire to prove one's merit. Growing up Catholic, Baptist, or Presbyterian, we aspire to be praiseworthy, follow the rules, and live a moral life. The desire to be unfailing and to receive approval from others is a powerful motivator. It dominates the sphere of private thoughts and influences every hope and fear.

The cleansing rituals that are integral to yoga provide just the right setting for these underlying aspirations to play out. Of course, not all yoga practitioners are prompted by this inner impulse. There are weekend warriors who go to yoga class to stay fit, socialize, find a date, or be part of the trend. But those who remain steadfast on the path for years, inspired to take a two-hundred-, five-hundred-, or one-thousand-hour teacher training program, may be compelled by what I think of as the demon of perfectionism.

I see the urge toward perfection played out in the yoga classroom all the time. Following the perfectionist's ideal, students believe that if they practice long and hard enough, they will come clean: they will purify, master, and align their bodies and be true. This determination runs parallel to the impulse to have a perfect body. I like to remind my students that there is no perfect pose;

rather, yoga is a process of being in the moment, moment by moment, while learning to accept limitations and accommodate pain and discomfort. Yet students are often motivated to prove themselves. They harbor unrealistic expectations of themselves and the practice. Exacting teachers who insist on the precise execution of a pose can exacerbate this tendency. This steals from the spirit of acceptance and prompts the student to a tireless pursuit of an unattainable ideal.

I have found that the yearning for perfection manifests in the classroom when considering the correct alignment of a pose. When students analyze a pose in training programs, there is often an underlying assumption that the body in yoga *should be* symmetrical. The body is not symmetrical. The liver is on the right, while the stomach is on the left; the left lung has two lobes, while the right lung has three. Breathing is not symmetrical because the diaphragm is a bit lopsided, or "wonky" (as they say in Britain). Nevertheless, students aspire to a perfectly balanced body. For instance, when learning a posture like warrior I pose, students ask, "Should my hips be square?" In this pose, the position of the right hip is not identical to the left, and the sacrum is slightly askew. In fact, there are real structural benefits to asymmetrical poses like warrior I, triangle pose (*trikonasana*), or revolved triangle (*parivrtta trikonasana*), given the way they effectively address strain and dysfunction in the body. Nevertheless, students get fixated on the idea that the hips in warrior I pose (and similar postures) be square. This is a real irony, for at the level of the fascia, joints, and organs, the body is asymmetrical. There are no straight lines in the human form. Yet the perfectionist craves exactitude and equal proportions, superimposing ideals of balance and symmetry onto organic structure. In pursuit of symmetry, the student sets up a binary of fulfillment versus failure. By positing the notion of balance and order, she strives for a hypothetical state of perfection, one that can never really be fully realized.

When I teach courses that include a detailed study of anatomy and structural alignment in yoga, I encourage teachers in training to acknowledge aberrations within their own structures. Everyone has a "signature shape." Our bodies are expressions of a multitude of historical forces that cause bones to torque, joints to rotate, and connective tissue to compress. We all have unilateral strain: one hip is higher than the other, or one shoulder is farther forward. None of us is symmetrical. One of my colleagues in Santa Fe, an osteopath named Don Smith, said that by the time we are twenty years old, we may have as many as fifty lesions (structural deviations) in the body. Falls, illnesses, and accidents give rise to our signature shape. The very emergence of life can precipitate structural imbalance, as in birth trauma during delivery. Yoga, qigong, osteopathy, Rolfing, and myofascial release should not endeavor to make the body perfect but rather support the body's signature shape.

While we address areas of somatic tension in order to mitigate dysfunction and move toward optimal health, acceptance of our signature shape promotes ease and well-being. When we acknowledge our asymmetries and accept the aberrations within our physical shape, we give up the ghost that craves perfect physical form. When we let go of the resolve to be perfect, we free up a tremendous amount of potential energy, because any preoccupation with impeccability requires significant mental and emotional effort to sustain.

Haunted by the demon of perfectionism, students can get obsessed with the sanitizing practices of yoga. Hatha yoga is essentially a codified system to purify the body. There are practices to flush the bowel, cleanse the gut, aerate the lungs, rinse the sinuses, enhance lymphatic drainage, polish the nerves, and clear the mind. Hatha yoga is a guide to total self-regulation: aspiring yogis regulate their diet, sleep, physical energy, sex drive, thoughts, and the very air they breathe. Dietary restrictions epitomize this: eating a vegan, vegetarian, or raw food diet can become a means to purify, cleanse, and control.

It is not only physical perfection that students are drawn to but also control of the mind. The mindfulness boom today is valuable as it encourages nonreactivity, consideration, and kindness. But for the perfectionist, mindfulness practice can intensify the urge to monitor. Meditation can become a project to control one's thoughts, desires, memories, and emotions. If mindfulness becomes all-consuming, it may result in hyper-conscientiousness. For the perfectionist who dreads making a mistake by hurting another person's feelings, or appearing selfish or out of control, mindfulness may become a spiritual rationale to fastidious and intense vigilance. On the Eightfold Path to enlightenment, the desire to do the right thing through right speech, right action, and right livelihood can trigger an obsessive urge toward perfection. This only chokes off the flow of the raw, potent, and creative force.

Growing up in middle-class America, it is implicit that each individual must perform well, get good grades, and stand on her own two feet. America is the land of "do it yourself." When strategies toward self-determination mix with Eastern practices espousing selflessness and unity, it can be confusing. It is telling that when the Dalai Lama first arrived in America from Tibet to share the teachings of Buddhism, the first thing he noted was that in America, the individual is vastly elevated. In the cultures of Tibet and India, the self is indivisible from the social fabric of family, school, and community. With the sense of selfhood always at stake, the motivation to receive approval, avoid criticism, and be successful looms large.

Under the sway of the demon of perfectionism, self-control is seductive. The student can get caught up in power struggles to achieve self-mastery. In fact, it is common for yoga studios and trainings to identify their guiding instructors as "master teachers." I always cringe to hear that phrase, for the notion that you can be master over your body or mind is completely far-fetched. If there is any mastery, it is the knowing that we are ultimately not in control. The path of yoga demands relinquishing the very notion of a fixed self-governing authority—an enduring, indestructible self. In fact, the path of yoga necessitates dismantling the seeming authority of self.

However, in the first half of the journey, students may become preoccupied with their own accomplishments in poses like handstand. The pursuit of mastery drives the longing for perfection deeper inside. Instead of pursuing mastery, we should seek mystery and the wild ways of grace, open to a force just beyond our grasp. This is difficult to do if we are consumed by an exacting desire to accomplish, achieve mastery, and become pure.

Today, cultural norms of the "body beautiful" impact the goals and desires of many yoga students. The longing to have a yoga body that is fat-free, light, and lifted motivates many to excel at practice. Women who compare their bodies to the slender figures of models on the runways are driven to pare down any extra flesh. In yoga classes today, populated mostly by women, there is a common aim to become featherweight and flexible. This gets exaggerated in studios with mirrors, where students spy on their fellow students and compare levels of physique and limberness.

The yearning to have a flat belly gets magnified by yoga techniques such as *bandhas*, *kriyas*, and the "breath of fire." In these practices, the abdomen is pumped, pulled inward, lifted, and churned. Traditionally these practices are cleansing techniques to purify the gut, increase digestive fire, and expand prana. Yet today, students mix yoga's purifying rituals with their own agendas to reduce body fat. Our culture's perception that to be beautiful, women must appear lithe and waif-like reinforces these efforts.

In yoga classrooms, the yearning for perfection may compound any tendency toward eating disorders. Yoga discipline that promotes dietary control, fasting, and lightness can be coupled with eating disorder. The desire to be faultless, to be perfect, and to realize the impossible goal of purity may become all-consuming. For those suffering from an eating disorder and the compulsion to have a clean and unsullied body, the demon of perfectionism is formidable.

The fear of shame motivates many to prove themselves in the world. Being deathly afraid of rejection and failure, we unwittingly side with the demon of perfection. The feeling of shame is crushing, and many go to extreme measures to be free from feelings of guilt, shame, and unworthiness. In yoga, it is often the power practices that push people beyond their limits. In these practices, stretching and strengthening the body may become self-punitive and exhausting. Students may rationalize doing severe and depleting practices under the guise of spiritual growth. If not pursuing physically rigorous practices, one may be self-condemning—denying themselves experiences of fulfillment and joy. Because the forces that motivate us to prove ourselves are so insidious and subtle, many of us unwittingly carry them out on the path of yoga.

Not all students on the path today undertake grueling practices. Inspired by an altruistic motivation, many devoted yoga enthusiasts bring yoga into prisons, recovery centers, and senior living facilities. But largely, yoga today is a means to self-improvement, prompting students to "reach their highest potential." In yoga circles there is a consensus that the primary aim of practice is self-renewal and that each of us must reconcile our own inner conflicts and work through our own karma. It is generally understood that each of us has to navigate our own inner demons. The primary means to accomplish this is self-restraint (*yama*). Yogis use rigorous discipline and control to overcome the "poisons," or obstacles, that inhibit progress on the path—namely, ignorance, fear, sexual craving, greed, and anger.

As we saw in the last chapter, attempts to realize right effort are often motivated by the ghosts of our Puritan forefathers. In the Judeo-Christian ethos, we are raised with clear dichotomies: good and evil, sacred and profane, sullied and pure. In the quest to sanitize purity and salvation, the motto "cleanliness is next to godliness" prevails. Generations that preceded us sought renewal and redemption by attempting to cleanse their homes and communities of the dark, the wild, the contaminated, the foreign, or the sinful. As a result, we live in a society that adheres to dualistic notions of male versus female, dark-skinned versus white-skinned, sanity versus insanity, and criminal versus innocent.

Our parents and grandparents—ministers, nurses, school-teachers, bankers, and builders—toiled through trials to live righteously. When I reflect on my own ancestry, I think of my grandmother, Virginia Little. I recall how fastidious she was in her kitchen, determined to set the table just right, keep the counters spotless, and do all the food prep herself. The kitchen was her domain, and I remember being scolded when I opened the refrigerator door. Currents of belief run deep through family lines, and we are each cut from a bolt of generations-long fabric. Each of us is influenced by the sensibilities, morals, and values of our family of origin. The idea that we incarnate out of previous lives is a longstanding cultural belief in India and throughout Asia. Whether or not you believe in reincarnation (certainly a slippery subject—topic for another book!), we are forged from the hopes, dreams, and fears of our parents and grandparents. We are shaped, quite literally, by the personalities that precede us.

The problem of purity and attachment to perfection in yogic discipline is not a new phenomenon. In the Great Way (Mahayana) record of Shakyamuni Buddha's teachings, the duality separating purity and pollution was carefully deconstructed. A collection of sutras called the *Maha Prajna Paramita* (*The Path of Great Wisdom*) includes instruction on the dangers of oppositional thinking, including the split between purity and impurity. In contrast to the long-standing belief that purity was essential to awakening, the Heart Sutra declares:

> . . . all dharmas are marked by emptiness
> they are neither created nor destroyed
> neither pure nor impure,
> they are neither complete nor deficient . . .[1]

The Heart Sutra points to a reality that transcends binary divisions. Cultures the world over have differing views about what qualifies as sanitary and pure. For instance, India, historically, has held stark views segregating the clean from the defiled. The caste system of India held to rigid divisions separating the pure from the polluted, defining an entire segment of the population as "untouchable." The priestly class, the Brahmins, were considered moral and virtuous, while people from the lower caste (typically tribal people of darker skin tone) were considered polluted. Dietary restrictions were carefully built into the caste system and it is well known that Brahmins historically would only eat food prepared by other Brahmins.

Adherence to firm convictions around sanctity and purity prompted a number of yogic sects to break away from rigid taboos. Sometimes called the "left-handed" path, yogis elected to eat meat, drink alcohol, engage in sexual relations, and practice in cemeteries. In one of his many guises, Siva appears as filthy, naked, and homeless. In the mythology of Siva, he appears as the "Supreme Beggar" (Bhikshatana) and challenges the righteous sensibility of the provincially minded sages.

Caution against prejudiced notions of purity and perfection is needed today as firmly held convictions around racial purity abound. For instance, the belief that people of color are inferior and that white supremacy should reign is a threat to the very fabric of our culture. The rise of the Third Reich in Nazi Germany and the eventuality of the Holocaust prove that convictions around racial purity lead to great danger.

By the time the Mahayana teachings on transcendental wisdom reached China and Japan, the troublesome divide between pure and impure, perfect and imperfect, had been carefully cautioned against. As a result, in the literature of China and Japan, a number of poignant passages dismantle the belief that purity is essential to enlightenment. This mischievous line from the celebrated Japanese

Zen poet Ikkyu suggests this: "That stone Buddha deserves all the birdshit it gets."[2] Following up with a similar view, the singer-songwriter and Buddhist maverick Leonard Cohen railed against excess piety and the obsession of the do-gooder when he wrote:

> Ring the bells that still can ring
> Forget your perfect offering
> There is a crack in everything
> That is how the light gets in.[3]

If left unchecked, the impulse toward perfection undermines spiritual growth. It limits a capacity to be kind, nonjudgmental, open, and carefree. It undermines the ability to find simple joy in the everyday. By accepting our own foibles and failures, we become more tolerant of ourselves and others. We stop trying to be someone else, someone more worthy, special, or enlightened. If we are not careful, the longing for perfection can close off the very source of light it is seeking.

PRACTICE, INQUIRY, AND REFLECTION

IN MEDITATION

Being with What Is

Sit in a comfortable position with your legs crossed, your spine upright, and your chest wide. Imagine that you are sitting in an old-fashioned beanbag chair so that the contact points of your sitting bones contour to the cushion below. Begin by taking several soft, slow breaths. Be aware of the movement of your breath. Do not attempt to manipulate your breath by making it bigger or longer. Observe your natural "breath print"; that is, yoke to the inherent motion of your respiratory rhythm. Watch your breath as if you are a neutral observer of your own vital force. Can you simply observe your breath rather than imposing an agenda to make it better?

In your meditation be accepting toward all that arises. As you settle in, become aware of any urge to perform the meditation correctly. Note any craving you may harbor to have perfect alignment in your body or to make your mind perfectly still. Make your concentration light and steady. Avoid micromanaging every breath, every thought, and every purpose. This steals from the spirit, and you are liable to get in your own way.

Reflect on how much energy, hope, and expectation you have invested in your efforts to become perfect over the years. How strong is the perfectionist streak inside you? Reflect on the ways you may have walked "a hundred miles through the desert" in order to gain approval, be liked, or deemed worthy. To what end? It is depleting and exhausting to be caught in the vise grip of perfectionism. Know that meditation is not a journey to become perfect or worthy in the eyes of God, family, or yourself. Rest assured that there is no bar for success in meditation that you need to reach. Let go of any preconceived idea that you must get the meditation right. Rather, be accepting toward all things that arise, whether pleasant or painful. Be kind to yourself by acknowledging your own imperfections. Let go of any notion of spiritual attainment or enlightenment. Reflect on the fact that any idea of perfection is just an idea. Rest in the living grace of the moment without the need to make it different than it is.

ON THE MAT

Your Signature Shape

Practice downward-facing dog pose. Start on your hands and knees with your shoulders aligned over your wrists. Look to your hands and stretch open your palms and fingers. Turn your hands slightly outward so that the webbing between your thumb and forefinger orients toward the top of your mat. Elongate your interior arms. Then lift back into the pose. Press your legs back away from your head. If you have tight hamstrings and lower-back muscles, bend your knees slightly. Be sure to release the weight of your skull so you are not straining your neck. Actively lift your shoulders. Once your pose is stable, observe your signature shape within the pose. As you bear weight into your wrists, elbows and shoulders, do the ligaments and tendons in one arm feel compressed? Do you feel one arm is shorter than the other? Or weaker? Does your signature shape cause one side of your lower back to pull more than the other? If you look at your feet in the pose, does one foot turn out more than the other? Where do you need to engage more, and where do you need to soften and spread? As you hold the pose longer, you will notice feelings of achiness, fatigue, and strain. Do you feel it more on one side than the other? Stay here for one to three minutes.

Transition to child's pose on the floor. Again, note your signature shape. Does one ankle feel more compressed? Do you have knee pain on one side more than the other? Breathe along the paraspinal muscles that flank your vertebral column. Does your breath feel more restricted on one side of your spine? Continue this process of observation throughout your practice. Over time you will have a clear internal sense of your signature shape.

OFF THE MAT

The Thief in the House

Become aware of the pressures you place on yourself to be perfect. In the course of a day, you may be compelled to get things right and appear good in the eyes of others. Note how often you get caught up in the urge to be flawless. Initially, this might involve your outward appearance. How often in a day do you feel displeased by the way you look? What expectations do you place on yourself regarding the appearance of your face, clothes, and hair? Be aware of the expectations you have of yourself in the role of student, parent, teacher, employee, or boss. Do those expectations cause strain or anxiety and eat away at your overall vitality? To what extent do you feel that you are always falling short, always less than?

Note how many times a day you compare yourself to others

regarding your looks, performance, and levels of success or popularity. If you are a parent, observe the expectations you harbor for your child. Are you imagining that she will be the very best in her field and earn millions of dollars? Be aware of the expectations you bring to your primary relationship with your husband, wife, or partner. Do you harbor ideals for your partner that are unrealistic?

Swept up in ideals of perfection, we are often overwhelmed and frustrated when plans go awry, mistakes occur, and life gets messy. Note the times when you get caught in cycles of blame, disappointment, and irritation because your expectations were not met. Note the places in your body where you clamp down and tighten as feelings of guilt, shame and unworthiness surface. How does it affect your jaw, neck, breath, or belly?

As you proceed through the course of your day, watch out for the demon of perfectionism. In Zen there is an expression: "It is hard to guard against a thief within." The urge to be perfect is likened to having a thief in your own house. When there is a thief in your house, it steals from your capacity to be accepting, at ease, and content. It may linger around you like a ghost, haunting your every move. A thief in the house always makes one feel afraid, restless, and unsettled. It may make you feel that things are never quite right and that you are responsible and at fault. An underlying feeling of dread creeps in, which only inhibits the expression of the creative spirit. On this day, note the occasions when you feel haunted by this thief, the demon of perfectionism. By acknowledging the presence of the demon, you cast light on the exaggerated expectations you place onto yourself. Have patience, kindness, and compassion toward yourself, toward others (especially those you live with) and too, have compassion for the demon trapped inside your house.

6

Not Knowing

IN INDIA EVERYONE loves babies. If you see a baby in a public setting, you will witness a throng of people cooing and clucking, entranced by the child-spirit. For the babe in Indian lore represents innocence, authenticity, and spontaneity. Within the plethora of gods and goddesses in India, one stands out as the most supreme and lovable. That is the enchanting, playful, flute-playing Krishna. This child-god is adored for his bounteous play and bliss-filled being and is a source of adoration in stories, myths, and temples. Like all children should be, he is mischievous, impassioned, irresistible, and fearless. In his charm and innocence, he embodies the essence of the absolute.

We could say that yoga is a rekindling of the heart of the child, for the spirit of the child is filled with awe and wonder. Unencumbered by the demands that plague adults, the child is connected to magic. The child revels in playful freedom, and the uncharted mind of the child is likened to a boundless, open presence. The child is easily absorbed, and his capacity to unequivocally be present is celebrated in yoga as a kind of *samadhi* (absorption). All the rituals of yoga—breathing practices, fasting, devotional offerings, and yoga *nidra* (meditative sleep)—invite a return to the unconditioned mind of the child.

At one time we all experienced the spacious awareness of the child, a state free from the polarizing limits of self versus other, inner versus outer, right versus wrong, and good versus bad. Inevitably when socialized, we break down the vast and immeasurable universe into small prefab boxes. This task, in large part, falls to our parents. As a parent myself, I found the responsibility of conditioning my child's reality daunting, guiding him from a state of unconditioned awareness to the importance of not throwing the butter knife at the dog or crawling around on the floor of the Whole Foods frozen food isle.

As a child, I was raised in part with lessons from the celebrated stars of *Sesame Street*—Big Bird, Grover, Ernie, and Bert. I distinctly remember as a budding five-year-old sitting in the big leather chair in our family den watching multiple episodes of this show. I witnessed bananas and oranges bounce across the screen in time to the little ditty, "One of these things is not like the other, one of these things just doesn't belong." Gazing wide-eyed at the screen, my unbounded mind was being indoctrinated, however melodiously and delightfully, into the ways of oppositional thinking.

One of the ways that we attend to the boundless, impartial realm of spirit is through not knowing. Not knowing involves witnessing impermanence, seeing that everything is like a river—fluid, ephemeral, and mercurial. Nothing can be nailed down. Everything is in flux, from the outermost galaxy down to the cells in your spleen. That everything is "fluxing," mutable, and uncertain lies at the heart of the Buddha's teaching on transience. Through a lifetime of practice, it is valuable to learn to accommodate uncertainty. How do you fare in the face of unpredictability and the unknown? Does it cause you to clench and tighten? To what extent do you feel the need to armor yourself against uncertainty in favor of temporary security?

Because things are inherently unstable, we never really know how they will go. When I awake each morning, I sit for a half hour in the space of not knowing. For that period of time I open myself up to possibility. I till the soil of my heart and mind, fertilize it with positive intention, and sit in the fertile ground of potentiality. I resolve to sit with a wide-open heart and alert mind, inhabited by space and clarity. In Zen, this state of mind is sometimes referred to as "radical openness." Zen master Shunryu Suzuki, author of *Zen Mind, Beginner's Mind*, described this simply, "Wisdom is a ready mind."

Despite my good intentions, there are times when I get tossed about in the throes of uncertainty. Pangs of fear creep in, anxiety crawls through my gut, and dread lodges in my shoulders and neck. Hesitancy and doubt metastasize quickly. When I struggle with uncertainty, I attempt to cultivate its antidote, fortitude, and trust. This is paradoxical. How can I live with confidence and resolve in the midst of an uncertain world? In the face of antipathy, violence, and prejudice, how do I remain open and receptive?

When our hearts crack open, at least a little bit each day, we feel more acutely the suffering inherent in being. A spark of loving-kindness ignites within the space of the rendered heart. This is what keeps the heart supple. Each morning, I rekindle an inner promise to stay fluid and receptive toward all that may come, whether painful or pleasant. In the midst of global uncertainties today, the path of radical openness is needed more urgently than ever before.

In the first half of practice, we tend to seek certainty. We believe unwaveringly in the code, the mantra, and the technique. For the many years that I did Ashtanga yoga, I held religiously to the sequence of postures that define the vinyasa practice. The structure and discipline of the form gave me the confidence and conviction to continue. I dove headlong into the practice, traveling to India to study, and as a result, the practice became my identity, my lifeline.

Having carried the staff of certainty for years and adhering closely to the formulas of practice, I eventually found a way to redefine my identity. Transitioning from a place of certainty and conviction to a place of not knowing is an arduous and daunting task. At some point, the spiritual path requires a leap into the unknown, outside the framework of the familiar. Moving into uncharted territory demands that we trust, have courage, and be willing to take a leap of faith. I am reminded of an old Chinese proverb, "To say you don't know is the beginning of knowing."[1] For me not knowing has opened up unforeseen vistas along the path.

When we relinquish having to know and open to something just outside our grasp, we enter a strange wonder, an anonymous space, full of mystery—the *magnum mysterium*. In the quiet hours when we rest in not knowing, stillness and peace bathe each and every cell and synapse of our being, and we connect to an energy source that sustains everything. In yoga the profound and immense energy that mothers all creation is called *shakti*. When we hush our conspiring, interpretive mind, we discover a latent, enduring energy. Like a prospector hitting a vein of crude oil under a layer of rock, we tap a tremendous current. It is through the power of not knowing that artists find inspiration, medical scientists conceive of new cures, and explorers reach new frontiers.

We never really know the outcome of what we do. For instance, not knowing is fundamental to the process of writing. As I compose this sentence, I follow the thread of not knowing. When you plant a garden, get married, or look up to the stars, you participate in the inscrutable ways of not knowing. Not knowing is the fuel, the raw energy that enables everything to move and shake.

The craft of teaching must include not knowing. I think the best teachers are those who have studied their material and can walk into a classroom in the spirit of not knowing, open to the way the class will unfold. Within any discipline, one must combine a learned familiarity with a willingness to embrace the unforeseen. Like a high-wire act, skillful action requires a tricky balance of knowing and not knowing, holding on and letting go, control and surrender.

Over time, we learn that not only are things unpredictable, but that we flourish precisely because they are indefinite. It is a paradox that the indefinite is the very ground of the infinite! In the way that we learn to ride a bike or drive a car, we learn to rely on the inconceivable; it becomes our means of transport. The inconceivable is extraordinary, a plenum of possibility, and when we learn to "ride" it, we are ferried along by its liberating presence. In the tribal cultures of Tibet, the wind horse symbolized the liberating spirit of the inconceivable, carrying on its back the prayers of the well-intended.

Not only is the great absolute a source of not knowing, but too, the smallest, most everyday phenomena is evidence of not knowing. The ordinary becomes a source of wonder when we realize that each passing thing is beyond knowing. Bashō, a master of haiku in seventeenth-century Japan, wrote,

> Morning glory!
> Another thing
> I will never know[2]

By the spirit of not knowing we experience the world as both beautiful and enigmatic.

The American Zen teacher Bernie Glassman identified not knowing as a central pillar of practice. He founded the Zen Peacemakers Organization and taught his students three fundamental tenets: not knowing, bearing witness, and taking compassionate action. Not knowing is a necessary first step on the journey; it is an invitation to suspend judgment, loosen fixed views, and live each moment open to possibility. For Glassman, not knowing is a means to return again and again to the ever-unfolding present. The second tenet, bearing witness, is an invitation to attend to each passing moment. In meditation, bearing witness is *vipassana*, "seeing into" all that arises. Inwardly, we start by noticing our breath, sensations, and meandering thoughts. By looking within, we bear witness to the maze of meanings we create. Outwardly, we perceive the world as a kaleidoscope of changing forms.

As witness, we are not separate, remote like a satellite observing from on high, but rather find ourselves smack-dab in the middle of circumstance. In the thick of our lives, we learn to witness and feel whatever is arising, whether pleasant, unpleasant, or neutral. We witness not only the harmonious and the sublime but also the mess, the hurt, and the longing. As a result, we build a kind of staying power to be with the trauma and the tears of our time. By acknowledging the pain of the world, we participate in the internet of being and grow more sympathetic, humane, and considerate. Glassman put it this way, "In Zen practice, we say that we do our sitting meditation not for ourselves but for the world."[3]

In the path of practice, wisdom does not come from mere intellectual study but rather from being a living testimony to loss and suffering. In order to embody the incalculable lament of the human soul, Zen Peacemakers Organization conducts retreats each year on the site of the Auschwitz-Birkenau concentration camp in Poland. There, people from all walks of life bear witness to the remnants of the engine of death. The practice includes sitting collectively in the midst of historical trauma. Retreat goers form a circle at the end of the rail track where the Nazi SS conducted their selections for the crematorium. A shofar is blown to start the meditation, and the names of those who were executed are spoken. Through this practice those bearing witness tune in to a living tremor of sorrow. Of the experience at Auschwitz, Glassman wrote:

> When we bear witness to Auschwitz, at the moment there is no separation between us and the people who died. There is also no separation between us and the people who killed. We ourselves, as individuals, with our identities and ego structure, disappear, and we become the terrified people getting off the trains, the indifferent or brutal guards, the snarling dogs, the doctor who points right or left, the smoke and ash belching from the chimneys. When we bear witness to Auschwitz, we are nothing but all the elements of Auschwitz.[4]

The last of the three tenets is compassionate action. There is nothing more pressing in the world today than rolling up our sleeves in service of the well-being of all. In the face of social injustice, environmental destruction, greed, and bigotry, compassionate action is imperative. When bearing witness, we behold the fragility inherent in being, and this prompts a spirit of kindness, care, and concern. When the embers of our hearts are stirred, we stand passionately for the truths in which we believe. Bearing witness allows us to respond without reactivity and vengeance but rather with *metta* (sympathetic kindness): *May all beings be free of physical, emotional, and psychological harm.* The great soul Mahatma Gandhi, marching against British rule in India in the 1940s, took action in the face of oppression, discrimination, and violence. He called his path *satyagraha*, or "holding to truth." Living satyagraha and taking compassionate action is instrumental to the path of yoga. Holding to the truths (*yamas*) of nonharming, honesty, nonstealing, abstinence from sexual misconduct, and generosity requires inner strength and a willingness to stand up against the vile front of misguided power.

Not knowing is a way to be more responsive, more alive, and more immediate. It frees us to be light on our feet. Not knowing allows us to be in the moment rather than operating from a preconceived notion about how things should be. If we have racing thoughts about the future, and are anxious and ridden with anticipation, it is hard to be genuine, dynamic, and responsive in each moment. While planning and strategizing have their place, overthinking causes the mind to pinwheel. Once in this mode, we can spin for hours. Caught by whirlwinds of anxiety and distress, we wake at 3 a.m. in spirals of thought. Yogis have known for centuries the dangers of obsessive thinking, that it burns the vital prana. Meditative awareness and deep silence slow the spin of thought.

Not knowing comes about through forays into unknown territory. Like a traveler in a foreign land, we shed the cloak of familiarity and experience the world afresh and new. As an example of this, the American poet Walt Whitman ventured across the backroads and urban streets of mid-nineteenth-century America. Raw, uncontrived, and curious, Whitman wandered in a spirit of revelation and discovery. Whitman, along with Ralph Waldo Emerson and Henry David Thoreau, was influenced by the Eastern ideals of introspection, liberation, and rhapsody. Having read the Upanishads and the Bhagavad-Gita, the Transcendentalists in New England were drawn to yoga metaphysics. In college, I was an avid reader of Whitman and his poetry inspired me to move outside the confines of my own small self. Always curious, always seeking, and ready to embrace a world teeming with difference, Whitman communed with soldiers, factory workers, immigrants, and moms alike. It was Whitman's "Song of the Open Road" that in part fueled my own passion for discovery, prompting me to roam the open roads of America, make a pilgrimage to India, and start on my yoga quest:

> From this hour I ordain myself loos'd of limits and
>   imaginary lines,
> Going where I list, my own master of total and absolute,
> Listening to others, considering well what they say,

pausing, searching, receiving, contemplating,
Gently, but with undeniable will, divesting myself of
the holds that would hold me.[5]

Full of sentiment, the path of not knowing makes the heart wide. Divested of its old predictable ways, the spirit within is made available, authentic, and clear. In each moment, we breathe in the miraculous display of the ever-changing world.

My teacher in the Dzogchen tradition of Tibetan Buddhism, Tsoknyi Rinpoche, underscores the importance of not knowing and what he calls "carefree dignity." Carefree dignity suggests an unconfined awareness, one that is not held back by mind-made limits and "imaginary lines." In meditation, not knowing is a doorway to nondual awareness. With our sitting bones on the cushion, each of us must come up against the suppositions and assumptions we harbor about ourselves and others. Endlessly productive, the ego concocts its own scenarios and scripts. It schemes and strategizes while trying to figure out just how to "do" meditation. However, meditation cannot be "done," for there is nothing to grasp or hold on to. Primarily, the practice is about divesting ourselves of the imaginary lines we draw in the sand of our minds.

In the Upanishads, not knowing was integral to liberated awareness along with mental absorption, selflessness, and nongrasping. The Mandukya Upanishad, recorded around the second century C.E., and influential in later formulations of Buddhist thought and practice, describes samadhi with real precision and depth. Following several verses elucidating the power of OM and descriptions of the three primary states of consciousness—waking, sleeping, and dreaming—the Upanishad describes a fourth state of deep peace. It is realized in the process of not knowing:

> Neither inside nor outside, incapable of being cognized, invisible, unspeakable, ungraspable, without any sign, unthinkable, unnamable, that in which the world comes to rest, peaceful and non-dual.[6]

This passage describes the state known as *prajna*, and we chose this very old word to represent our school in Santa Fe, New Mexico: Prajna Yoga. It is akin to the Greek word *gnosis* and is related to the bizarre spelling of the English word *knowledge*. Yet prajna is not the kind of knowledge you gain when you memorize your times tables or learn the capitals of countries. Prajna is a much stranger knowing. It is untenable, always eluding the configuring ego. Slippery and subtle, this knowing is paradoxically not knowing. Thus in meditation, any accumulation of knowledge is a sure sign of trouble. As soon as you think you have it, you are hundreds of miles off course. Whatever is grasped or gotten in yogic meditation inevitably conforms to the ego's own likeness. We have the expression in English "It's not what you think," a turn of phrase that applies aptly to yogic wisdom. It is most confounding that enlightenment requires not getting, not seeing, not possessing, and not knowing.

On the first part of our journey, we are eager to do practices that boost our identity. We may assume a Sanskrit name, follow a guru, become devoted to a specific style of practice, or travel to India. We take on an identity that feels more worthy than our former myopic, preoccupied self. This provides a needed foothold on the path to self-improvement. It lays the groundwork for the second phase of practice, when we proceed to unravel the very notion of self. We realize that the self I assume to be me is not so substantial. Through rigorous investigation into the nature of self, we come to see that the self is more vapor than solid. Like clouds that come together for a brief period of time before dissolving, the self is a temporary accumulation. It is a cluster of impressions, ideas, memories, and reflections.

The German philosopher Immanuel Kant shared the Mahayana vision, suggesting that things are inherently unknowable, while being "things-in-themselves." He wrote, "I have no knowledge of myself as I am, but merely as I appear to myself."[7] In the age of iPhones, screen sharing, and "selfies," the self is outwardly reinforced. There is nothing inherently wrong with the proliferation of the self through photos and the like, for the self has always been an appearance. When we realize that there is no solid "I" to be known, that no reasoning will elucidate the self and we cease any attempt at trying to find it, we open ourselves up to a universe of possibility. In this way we move from the personal to the transpersonal, from "me" to "we," and from the universe to the "Buddhaverse."

PRACTICE, INQUIRY, AND REFLECTION

IN MEDITATION

Not Knowing—The Highest Wisdom

Begin in a seated position that is stable and comfortable. Prop your pelvis up in such a way that you do not accumulate strain in your feet, knees, or hip joints. Take the first five minutes to settle into the bones at the foundation of your pose. Cultivate heaviness at your base while simultaneously stretching your spine vertically upward. Sense that the intervertebral discs between your spinal bones are buoyant. Float the back of your skull upward as if there is a small pocket of helium between your occiput and your first cervical vertebra (atlanto-occipital joint). Steady your concentration on the rise and fall of your breath. Nurture an embodied presence, one that is grounded, open, and full of ease.

Next, bring your awareness to the transient thoughts that surface in your mind. You will likely recognize excerpts from the script of your day in the form of bits of conversation, concerns, ideas, and obligations. Snippets of songs, little ditties, may waft through your head. Note the way that all mental stimuli drift through your awareness like passing clouds. Recognize each thought to be an excerpt of your personal narrative. All that appears on the screen of your awareness is part of the landscape of "you." By recognizing bits of memory, shards of thought, and fragments of belief, you travel the pathways of the familiar. Note your thoughts while reducing your mind's tendency to pinwheel round and round.

Now shift your awareness to that which you do not and cannot know and rest for a time outside the constraints of recognition. Come to this awareness by resting in the space between thoughts. Like the silence that accompanies musical notes, the emptiness at the top of an hourglass, or the empty space in the middle of the classic Zen circle, called the *enso,* this is a place of pure potential. While in this space, remind yourself that you do not need to know. All thoughts, ideas, or concepts are the domain of the limited, prescribed you. By shifting perspective to an open-ended awareness, outside the demarcation lines of identity, abide in not-knowing. Relinquish any attempts to know. Slow down your experience further by noticing the quality of awareness in the empty space of not knowing. Does it feel quivery, solid, luminous, or expansive? What is your relationship to silence and stillness? Do you feel a shift in your respiratory rhythm, blood pressure, and intracranial space?

Thoughts will likely surge back, vying for your attention. The contours of the ego-self will attempt to colonize the open, liberated space of not knowing and lay claim. Witness again the familiar domain of thought, perception, and belief. Then return, through the portal of perception, into a space of not knowing. Sense for a time the raw, embryonic potency of this space, free of motive and full of potential.

ON THE MAT

Standing Still, Traveling Far

This practice involves the simple art of standing. The following position is the first posture of qigong practice. It builds the resolve and concentration of the hunter as it brings steadfast calm to the nerves, enduring strength to the bones, and clarity to the heart and mind.

Stand with your feet slightly wider than hip-width apart. Bend your knees so they are both supple and strong. Distribute your weight evenly through the bones of your feet. Allow the weight of your tailbone to descend like a stalactite growing downward from the roof of a cave. Simultaneously float your spine upward like a column of steam. Be sure that your spine is balanced along its central axis—that is, avoid your spine cantilevering forward or backward. Sense and feel the deep life force that travels through your spine.

Set your hands in a circular position just in front of your navel, palms facing one another. Keep your fingers and wrists open but soft, as if there are bands of light shooting out from your fingertips. The spherical shape that you form with your hands and arms suggests the Zen circle, the enso. Let your posture be natural, fluid, and bold. The qigong master and martial artist Wang Xiang-zhai (1885–1963) taught that the secret of standing is emptiness. He wrote, "In movement, be like the dragon and tiger. In stillness, have the mind of the Buddha."[8]

Do not control your breath; rather, observe the way your qi courses through your bloodstream and along your nerve channels. Breathe in such a way that your breath billows into your kidneys. In Chinese medicine and qigong, the kidneys are the reservoirs of the body's vitality. Initiate lift in your L2 and L3 vertebrae, at the level of your kidneys. Here is located *ming men*, the "gate of life" acupuncture point. Ming men is responsible for qi flowing through the kidneys and it is the source of the long river of the spine.

After three to five minutes, straighten your legs and sense your internal pulses. Be aware of any small shifts in your blood pressure, respiratory rhythm, and circulatory flow. Take your stance three-six inches wider and bend your knees again, this time sinking lower toward the earth. Assume the same position with your hands. In the spirit of not knowing, bring a sense of curiosity and wonder to your practice. As you build staying power, bear witness to the sensations in your connective tissues through your arms, spine, legs, and feet. Observe the electrical flow through your skin, fascia, muscles, and bones. Observe the flow of sensations in your body, whether pleasant or painful. Remain for five to ten minutes, per your capacity.

OFF THE MAT

Not Knowing, Bearing Witness, Expressing Compassion

As you begin your day, invoke the spirit of receptivity, open-mindedness, and not knowing. Be prepared to meet each passing circumstance with a spirit of discovery and surprise. Reflect on how it is not possible to know exactly how circumstances will unfold. How can you predict the spin of time? All too often we feel like we should know how things will go, as if living is a follow-the-dots exercise. As you proceed with your plans for the day, give yourself the space and freedom not to know how events will transpire. This is not an easy practice because all too often, we set expectations for how things "should" happen. As you go move through your day, stay flexible, adaptable, and alert.

When you mindfully approach your day in a spirit of not knowing, what changes occur internally? Do you feel trepid and nervous, or do you feel enlivened, open to possibility? Within the spirit of not knowing, bear witness to all that may arise inside you. Are there instances when you feel anxious, restless, or impatient? Or do stronger emotions arise such as anger, hatred, or jealousy? Observe the shifting attitudes, moods, and tensions in your body.

At the same time, bear witness to the ever-changing world around you. That everything is changeable and uncertain lies at the heart of the Buddha's teaching. As you bear witness to time passing, note the thread of suffering that weaves through the lives of family members and friends. Recall that in bearing witness, we become a living testimony to the pain of the world. Bearing witness is not distance learning. It suggests that we are participants in the anguish, the joy, and the folly of the world.

The Tibetan meditation adept Lama Mipham wrote, "Contemplate to capacity all the pain of the human condition."[9] Not only do we recognize the suffering of the human condition but also the frailty of the insects, the plight of endangered species, and the loss of the ocean habitat. When we witness the exquisite beauty of the world on fire, we feel both joy and pain in the sinews of our hearts.

In this practice you need not resolve or fix anything; simply behold and "take to heart" all that surfaces during the course of today. When we bear witness and take things to heart, we feel tender, grateful, and kind. Bearing witness implies a kind of detachment—not a cold, remote detachment, but an impartiality that is both generous and warm. Welcome all that arises with equanimity. Equanimity implies the strength to embrace what happens. Through compassionate action, generate kindness and care toward all things.

7

The OM Shanti Experience

IN ALMOST EVERY yoga class today, the teacher will inevitably say something like, "Let your heart be open" or "Experience joy of being" or "Have gratitude for each moment." Verbal instructions bid students toward an experience of light and love. The underlying suggestion is that to embody the true state of yoga, you must feel sanctity, delight, and harmony. Yoga is equated with OM *shanti*, a feel-good experience that guides us to higher connection with the "true" self. Classes that pipe in upbeat vibes, ranging from techno bhakti grooves to old-time rock 'n' roll, transport the student to exulting states. All practice is meant to lead to the body of bliss.

Undoubtedly these platitudes are well-intentioned, and there are real benefits in propagating messages that promote positive, optimistic, and cheery dispositions. Yet the descriptions of the feel-good state can be misleading. It is naive to think that any of us can abide in a state of continuous bliss. To be fully human is to experience a full spectrum of emotions. This inevitably includes feeling the blues, feeling ambivalence, or just feeling "bent out of shape." In the same way that we build range of motion in the body, so we build range of emotion. By attending to the vicissitudes of sentiment, mood, and feeling, we build emotional intelligence.

Why has yoga come to be equated with a state of nectarine sweetness? What has inspired yoga to be a practice of good vibes promoting *irie* feelings and OM shanti revelry? In so doing, what may be neglected, overlooked, and ignored? The notion of the bliss-filled body is reflected in some of the earliest yoga teachings that chart the body-mind matrix as a series of sheaths or layers (*koshas*). The super-fine, inner most layer, the *ananda kosha*, suggests a state of superlative delight, specifically via unification with the Supreme Spirit. The notion that yoga is a bliss-filled state is certainly an attractive one, enticing students toward an experience of happy body and happy mind.

I am all for experiences that promote well-being and a positive outlook. However, as a collective we are wont to ignore painful or conflicted feelings and default to modes of feeling good. Our culture favors the application of the smiley emoji after each message. We are quick to gloss over feelings of angst and sorrow: when asked, "How are you?" our typical response is "Fine" or "Good." There is an implicit consensus that everyone should appear content, and if you don't, you are not living up to the status quo.

The writer Kate Bowler identified the perils of having to feel good as the "tyranny of prescriptive joy."

I have concerns that yoga students, desirous of equanimity, unwittingly become confined by this tyranny, duped into believing that they ought to be content all the time. If misinterpreted, yoga becomes equated with an untroubled and unruffled disposition. If a yogi is biased toward the sweet state, he risks paving over feelings of pain and sorrow.

In my first years of my practice, I used yoga as a kind of sedative. By riffing through multiple gravity-defying poses, I became adept at putting myself into a very pleasant stupor. After two hours of vigorous practice, I felt suspended in a cloud of bliss. The feeling was delightful and admittedly preferable to the gnawing angst that would often take hold of me. Through practice I learned to put myself under a kind of spell, a perfectly benign state free from affliction. I was convinced at the time that this self-imposed state was the dispassionate, unflappable joy espoused by the yoga scriptures. However, I discovered, to my dismay, that the serene sheen of my post-yoga state would inevitably wear off. When stranded in traffic, quibbling with my wife, or being ignored by my ten-year-old son, I would feel irritable and restless. When the aura of rapture wore off, I always felt disheartened. After so much yoga, I wondered, *Why is this happening?*

In the first years of practice, we may use yoga as a positive substitute, paving over conflicted feelings in order to feel lighter and uplifted. This works for a time and enables many of us to sidestep darker and more conflicted states of depression, anger, craving, or doubt. However, in the second phase of my yoga practice, I stopped using yoga to blunt the edge of my feelings. Instead, I used the practice to enhance my connection to a wide range of emotional states.

A forerunner in the field of psychology, mysticism, and dream work, Carl Jung practiced yoga. In his investigations into the psyche, Jung was profoundly influenced by Indian mythology, art, and symbolism. However, he practiced yoga carefully and with discrimination. In his autobiography, *Memories, Dreams, Reflections*, published in 1965, he describes his experience with yoga,

> I was frequently so wrought up that I had to eliminate the emotions through yoga practices. But since it was my purpose to learn what was going on within myself, I would do them only until I had calmed myself and could take up again the work with the unconscious.[1]

It is not known precisely what postures or pranayama practices Jung adopted, except that he practiced a kind of savasana. When lying down he would attune to his breath, bodily sensations, moods, memories, and, of course, dreams. (Similarly, Sigmund Freud elected to have his clients lie on a couch when under analysis.) I return to the importance of savasana in the last chapter of this book, but suffice to say here that should you wish to plumb the interior layers of your body-mind, awareness must be made receptive. While a vigorous yoga practice can ward off the ghosts and demons lurking in the psyche for a time, a slow and tactful practice infused with deep listening enables you to investigate the multiple and complex layers of self.

When penetrating the many layers of textured feeling, we delve into the subtle body. This includes noting the way anxiety lodges in the diaphragm, the way fear knots the solar plexus, or the way feelings of self-condemnation harden the delicate tissues of the throat. In subtle body awareness we note changes in blood pressure, heart rate, neurological impulse, and gut tension. This process makes available nuanced perceptions and sensations that were previously inaccessible. In this light, pranayama and postural practices are not intended to simply amp up the body in order to make it more flexible and stronger. Rather, we learn to observe the way sentiment manifests in the body—what Candace Pert called "the molecules of emotion." Through increased sensory aware-ness, we explore the understory of "self" and connect to the feeling states that determine all mood, attitude, thought, and behavior.

Many of us have a kind of sweet tooth: we prefer pleasure to pain, lightness to dark, shanti to struggle. We are creatures that default to "cozy-wozy" feelings any chance we get. If we are not careful, we may sugarcoat our experience. We may don a mask to appear positive and upbeat but, in so doing, run the risk of denying difficult and complex feelings. Should feelings arise that are antithetical to a yogic state of equanimity, we sweep them under the rug in favor of outer composure. This sets up a kind of dissonance and makes authentic response to the trials and tribulations of the world difficult.

To be authentic, honest, and, "real," it is important that we embrace our own shortcomings, foibles, and failures. The poet W. H. Auden famously wrote, "Love your crooked neighbour / With your crooked heart." By acknowledging feelings of anxiety, fear, sorrow, or confusion, we come to accept our humanity. In this regard, yoga is not an extraordinary state, one in which we transcend a capacity to feel but rather a practice to "be with" ordinary feeling states. This leads to greater sensitivity, tenderness, and humility. It is the very source of loving kindness.

Throughout a lifetime each of us experiences gain and loss, joy and sorrow, birth and death. Rather than opting for the OM shanti experience, we learn to accept the troubling and the uplifting, the bitter, and the sweet. Great feeling is inspired within us when we acknowledge the fragility of all things: our little blue earth spinning through space, the call from a grade-school friend not heard from in years, the wide open eyes of a darling pet, the podcast interview with the young mother who has since died of cancer at age thirty-eight. Each moment is tinged with a kind of sorrow, grace, and wistful appreciation.

One of my teachers tagged the compound word "joy-pain" when describing the admixture of grace and sorrow. This is suggested in Chinese medicine, wherein the heart is the center of joy, and the lungs are receptacles of grief and sadness. Anatomically, the lungs and heart are enmeshed, woven together by the stout pulmonary arteries and veins. In the very air that flows through the intricate network of the heart and lungs, "joy-pain" circulates.

It is by walking the path of pain that we open up vistas within our interior landscape that were previously obscured from view. We begin by learning to accommodate pain in our musculoskeletal system. Practicing yoga postures instigates some degree of pain in our fascia. We explore the edge of pain by stretching muscle, tendon, bone tissue, and joint capsule. We refer to the healthy mobilization of constricted fascia as "good pain." Learning to accommodate physical pain is an important first stage on the path. When attentive to our own physical discomfort, we learn to be with our "pain body." If unable to attend to our pain body, we often default to "rejecting mind"—denying, resisting, or feeling frustration toward our bodily experience. It is critical today that people gain tools to manage their pain and discomfort, as our medical industry is swamped with those who are unable to cope with pain. The opioid crisis that has ravaged America in past years and left so many people addicted to painkillers suggests the need for people to engage their body of pain.

In the second tier of yoga practice, we learn to accommodate heart pain and "mind pain." While many yoga practitioners are game to work deeply in their hamstrings or hip joints, many are reluctant to stretch into the dark spaces of the psyche.

Jung coined this "shadow work," and it involves reckoning with the vital energy of the demon. In the mythology of India and the archetypal realm of the psyche, the beneficent does not exist without the dreadful, nor does delight exist without disgust. When ready, and when we have support of a therapist or guide, we make a vertical descent into the shaded side of our psyche. When Theodore Roethke writes, "In a dark time, the eye begins to see," he suggests that the dark is both fertile and necessary. In order to navigate the dark thickets of shame, repression, or angst on the spiritual quest, we all pass through a "dark night of the soul." How do we learn to travel in the dark? Wendell Berry, a farmer poet from Kentucky, wrote:

> To go in the dark with a light is to know the light.
> To know the dark, go dark. Go without sight,
> and find that the dark, too, blooms and sings,
> and is traveled by dark feet and dark wings.[2]

How do we incorporate our shadow into the vision we hold of ourselves?

Given the tenuous turn in this part of the path, a counselor, shaman, guru, or guide is necessary. When passing from the well-lit world of Facebook and the snapshots of the social self to the hidden, murky realm of the dark, we cannot go solo; we must be led by someone who has made the crossing before us. Inevitably we feel disoriented, vulnerable, and trepid. In the face of uncertainty, we must risk putting our trust in another. We must renounce our former self and learn to trust the path in front us. Most never let their guard down enough to give themselves over to trust. They would rather stay in the light where everything appears solid and familiar. However, the umbra is the very source of visions, dreams, and intuitive knowing. One of my Zen teachers, Roshi Joan Sutherland, called the time in communion with the unknown "the process of endarkenment." In traveling the road to enlightenment, we must be willing to traverse dark trails that lead through strange and uncharted landscapes.

Great fortitude and courage is needed. When traipsing into unknown territory, we invoke the valor and strength of the archetypal warrior. In yoga posture, the prowess of the warrior is repeated in standing lunges (such as warrior pose), combining the grace of the Renaissance fencer and the mettle of the Japanese samurai. However, the warrior is too often confused with might and rule and the subjugation of energy. While the physical warrior is characterized by virility, the verve of the spiritual warrior is humility. In the healing arts, the true warrior is the wounded warrior, who emerges from the shadows having integrated his or her trauma and pain. The tenderness and sensitivity required to heal another is contingent on first having walked through the valley of loss and suffering.

In the Buddhist view, compassionate understanding is born from the direct experience of suffering. This was the experience of the young prince Siddhartha Gautama, who was born into a noble family in the fourth century B.C.E. in present-day Nepal. His mother died seven days after his birth, and he was raised by his aunt and well-to-do father. At the age of twenty-nine, he left the comfortable confines of his father's palace, only to witness a sea of suffering. He encountered the cries of the hungry, the pain of the infirm, and the mental anguish of the tormented. It was this direct experience of suffering that set him on a quest to discover an antidote to affliction. In the first formulation of the Buddha's teaching following his awakening, he described four essential "truths" about the human experience: (1) all sentient beings suffer physical, emotional, and psychological hardship; (2) suffering is caused by craving and clinging to a fleeting world; (3) craving is not inherent and can be remedied; and (4) there is a way to alleviate suffering, the Eightfold Path. In the Buddha's vision, pain is inherent in being. The wandering Japanese Zen poet Bashō captured the existential suffering of the world in this way:

> Come, see
> Real flowers
> Of this painful world.[3]

In the first half of my journey, I was more concerned with avoiding suffering than meeting it. I naively thought that if I practiced long enough and hard enough, I would become immune to pain and confusion. I was repeatedly disappointed when my old demons would tug at me, for I thought the state of yoga involved rising above distress and uncertainty. In the beginning of my practice, I was like a moth attracted only to light. Looking back, I see that the healing I did in the first half of my journey was preparatory for going further into the dark—into fear, shame, and the strange ways of the soul's own healing. This required embracing both the light and the dark. To live openly with fierce authenticity requires a willingness to sense and feel not only the sweet and the shanti, but the mucky, distasteful, and terrifying.

Peter Levine, in his groundbreaking work on trauma and recovery, wrote, "Body sensation, rather than intense emotion, is the key to healing trauma."[4] As we begin to sense and feel more, we wake up parts of ourselves that have been asleep or frozen. The process of unthawing can cause strange and prickly sensations. As we slough off old cells and prana comes back to areas that have been shut down and constricted, we feel more alive. Jane Hirshfield captured this process of waking in a poem from her collection *Given Sugar, Given Salt*:

Even now,
decades after,
I wash my face with cold water—

Not for discipline,
nor memory,
nor the icy, awakening slap,

but to practice
choosing
to make the unwanted wanted.[5]

In the same way that making the hamstrings longer and the hip joints more flexible requires time and persistence, learning to accommodate the unwanted requires practice. While the first years of yoga training are more geared to mellowing and composing the body-mind and generating positive sensory input to heal, in time we learn to integrate that which was forgotten, dismissed, or repressed. We no longer simply seek out the OM shanti experience, but by making the unwanted wanted, we revive crucial parts of ourselves that have been ignored, forgotten, or dismissed.

PRACTICE, INQUIRY, AND REFLECTION

IN MEDITATION

Sitting with Both Pain and Joy

This meditation involves sitting with feelings of conflict or loss while at the same time feeling support, trust, and guidance. Start by sitting comfortably on your cushion. Rest your hands, palms down, on your upper thighs so your hands are wide and soft. Lift your spine like a tree growing toward the light. At the same time release your shoulder blades down your back. Release the weight of your jaw and allow your tongue to rest behind your lower teeth. Make your eyes very soft and gel-like. Cast your gaze softly downward toward your heart and lungs. Become aware of your breath. Be sure that it is natural, rhythmic, and spontaneous.

While continuing to keep your right palm grounded on your thigh, turn your left palm upward. Allow the skin of your palm and fingertips to be open and receptive. Then bring to mind a positive force in your life. It can be a god, grandparent, teacher, friend, pet, or place that is an unconditional support for you in your growth and healing. Visualize a positive, luminous presence in your left hand, wrist, arm, and shoulder. Allow this presence to infuse your left lung and heart with light. Then turn your left palm back down to your thigh once again and sense the stability of your sitting bones, legs, and hands.

Now turn your right palm up toward the sky, resting the back of it on your thigh. Be receptive through the tips of your fingers and the skin of your palm. Bring to mind a circumstance, relationship, or memory that is a source of conflict or hardship for you. Avoid plummeting into the "center of the cyclone"; instead, mindfully tune in to some pain or sorrow that you have previously experienced. Alternatively, you might bring to mind the anguish and suffering of someone or something outside yourself. Just touch the edge of the shadow of your pain body. Note the sensations in your right hand, wrist, arm, and shoulder. Without judging or attempting to reconcile the painful feeling, allow yourself to be touched delicately and deeply by the pain. Notice any sensations that travel through your right lung and shoulder. Once the feeling of loss, sorrow, or pain moves through you, turn your right palm back down to your thigh. Sense the stability of both of your hands and feel your legs connected to the floor.

Now turn both hands upward at the same time and rest the back of your hands on your thighs. Simultaneously bring to mind the support of the positive presence on your left side and the feeling of conflict or tension on your right side. Be curious as you welcome both the unconditional support together with your body of pain. Trust that you can hold space in your body and mind for both joy and pain. Then bring your palms together in the gesture of *namaste* consolidating the forces of light and dark, joy and sorrow, love and fear.

ON THE MAT

Spinal Wave

Begin by lying on your back on a carpet or on a blanket spread over your sticky mat. Prior to moving, scan your entire body, and with a global awareness: feel your neck, chest, belly, and pelvis. What sensations can you notice within? Do you feel any discomfort, constriction, pain, or achiness? What does the discomfort feel like? Is the sensation prickly or sharp, dull or expansive? How much fatigue do you hold in your body? Note the rise and fall of your breath. Then sense your heartbeat in the left side of your chest. Bring awareness to the pulses in your hands, wrists, and forearms. Note any electrical tingles or murmurs of sensation in your neck and skull.

Bend your knees and set your feet hip-width apart on the floor. Take your arms out to your sides. Rock your pelvis into an anterior tilt as you inhale, arching your lower back. Be sure that your pelvis maintains contact with the floor. Then scoop your pelvis into a posterior tilt as you exhale, thereby rounding your lower back. Continue tilting back and forth, combining your breath with the movement. On each inhalation, breathe into your abdomen. Allow your belly to expand and widen as you arch your lumbar spine. With each exhalation, empty your abdomen by rounding your lower back and pressing it to the floor. Visualize your abdomen like a tide pool, filling on the in-breath and emptying on the out-breath. Note any sensations that arise in your skin, fascia, organs, or bones as you do this movement.

Then move your cranium in a similar rocking motion. Keep your head in contact with the floor, tuck your chin toward your sternum and arch your lower back—all on inhalation. As you round your lower back and breathe out, rock your chin upward toward the ceiling. Articulate the movement of your neck and lower back together in this breathing pattern. Note the feeling of a wave-like flow through your spine. Repeat six to ten of these spinal waves, and then stretch your legs out straight on the floor.

Note the way your bones drop into the floor. Scan your body again. Does it feel different than when you first lay down? Sense any small shifts in the rhythm of your breath and any nuanced changes in your interior pulses. Scan your body for any constriction, pain, or tension. Note the areas where your body feels light, spacious, and at ease.

OFF THE MAT

Feeling into Dreams

In both Western psychology and yoga, investigating the landscape of dreams has been instrumental to the process of navigating the shadowy underworld of the psyche. Patanjali, in the Yoga Sutras, points out that by reflecting on dreams, the practitioner gains insight (*jnana*) in preparation for yogic absorption (samadhi). The following dreamwork practice involves dream recall, exploring the sensory content associated with dream images.

We all have dreams that dramatize love, anxiety, fear, shame, ecstasy, and loss. While dream scenarios may appear bizarre and off-putting, consider that dreams simulate unexpressed feelings. In this regard, circumstances within dreams dramatize latent mind states. Dream recall provides an opportunity to access sensations and feelings that have been avoided, covered up, or otherwise made unavailable to us in the waking state. When working with dreams, we explore how the sensory content of a dream impacts our subtle body.

For example, I once had a dream where I was rushing to catch an airplane. The lines were long, and when I looked at my watch, I realized that the plane was about to leave. I felt stranded and at a loss. On reflection, I invoked the feeling of standing in line at the airport with a feeling of dread and anxiety. I recalled the sinking feeling of helplessness from the dream, noticing how the feeling caused a clenching in my gut and constriction in my ribs. Slowly and mindfully I acknowledged the feeling of constriction. By invoking the scenario within the dream that prompted the anxiety inside me, I could bear witness to my own state of internal tension. As it turns out, this anxiety was familiar, but it was one that I typically avoid at all costs.

In this practice you can be sitting quietly or lying down. Start by establishing connection to the ground below you and sense the rise and fall of your breath. Take the first five minutes to come to open presence. Then recall an image from one of your dreams that provoked a strong feeling. Evoke the image by selecting it as an object for your meditation. Observe the impact the image has on your subtle body. What sensory impressions does the dream image evoke? Do you feel constriction, irritation, a fluttering, or expansion? How does it feel in your jaw, throat, or gut? How does recalling the image affect your breathing? Do you feel pressure in your head, or do you feel light-headed and spacey? Avoid trying to interpret what the dream means or figure out why you had it. Avoid judging the content of your dream as good or bad.

As you acclimate to the feelings invoked by the dream image, notice any alchemical shift in your subtle body. By acknowledging the presence of a dream image and focusing on it as an element in your meditation, tension states within you will gradually shift. Note if places of holding loosen their grip. By acknowledging the undertow of feelings associated with dream scenarios and bringing them to light, we touch into the very source of a rich emotional life.

8

In the Flow of Presence

AS WAYFARERS ON the path, we travel many miles. We trek through thick forests and icy fjords, over rock-strewn terrain and desert wasteland. We may find ourselves inspired, bored, curious, or hungry. We may feel centered and at peace inside, or we may feel discombobulated and lost. More than likely, the long circuitous trail we are traveling will leave us exhausted and in need of rest. Whatever turn we take on the trail, whatever scenery we encounter, whatever our state of mind, the path we travel is designed to lead us to where we are right now.

Being on the path is a practice in presence. We start by feeling our feet contour to the ground, the weight of our knapsack and the rise and fall of our breath. We come into the flow of presence, a presence that lifts us and carries us on, like a four-year-old held high on the broad shoulders of his father. When we are present, we are suspended on the stream of time. We follow the course of flow and trust in its direction.

The flow of presence has been celebrated in China since the sixth century B.C.E., as an expression of the movement of the Tao. The flow of Tao is likened to the flow of water. Like a waterway that moves incessantly, the Tao is without fixed principles, always changing and responsive. Water always flows relative to its surroundings: stones, stumps, and riverbanks guide its course. In mountain glades where its path is steep and rock-filled, the river's current is swift and turbulent; in the broad plains where the river is wide and deep, its progress is slow and unhurried. "It is thus that Tao is like a river flowing down the valley to the ocean," said Lao Tzu in the *Tao Te Ching*.[1] The most important thing to remember is that we are always in the watery presence of now.

This is a presence much greater than ourselves, yet it always includes us. In the way that a fish makes its home in water or a bird travels through air, we are never apart from it. For this reason it is said in the Chinese classic *The Doctrine of the Mean*, "The Tao is that from which one cannot deviate; that from which one can deviate is not the Tao."[2] This ever-present Tao is all around us and inside every molecule and atom of our beings. In quantum physics, it is the ever-present field, the all-containing background, while simultaneously the dance of the smallest particle. Any observer who attempts to detect her exact location encounters real difficulty. While we are always a part of the flow of presence, we cannot pinpoint it—never mind acquire it, brand it, or call it our own. Presence is puzzling. It is difficult to catch, for presence is a fleeting thing:

> The Tao of Heaven operates mysteriously and secretly;
> it has no fixed shape; it follows no definite rules; it is so
> great that you can never come to the end of it; it is so deep
> that you can never fathom it.[3]

If the path of practice is to be in the now, how do we realize it? How can we grasp that which has no fixed shape and follows no definite rules? How do we live a life of presence in tune with our surroundings?

Players of all disciplines crave immersion in the moment. Saxophonists, figure skaters, the center fielder for the Boston Red Sox, Zen calligraphers, and tai chi masters alike relish the opportunity to become absorbed in their craft. Yogis look for the experience of absorption *all the time.* They are not content to experience isolated and short-lived states of absorption. If the process of absorption is limited to the ninety minutes we spend on our three-by-eight sticky mat each day, then the process of yoking is only partial. The aim of practice is ongoing, total 24/7 immersion. How is this possible?

For the majority of people, the experience of absorption is rare. It comes and goes. Only in sleep, at the movies, during sex, or under the influence of alcohol do people feel rapture. More often, they feel fragmented and distracted, anxious and overwhelmed.

Rather than feeling suspended on the current of the river of now, they feel like they are paddling hard upstream, getting pushed sideways, or pulled under.

In the way that an artisan would spend hours on a stone or wooden sculpture—chiseling, sculpting, shaving, whittling, and brushing—yogis hone the art of being in the present moment. When practicing a yoga posture, our bodies are the medium we work in: muscle, bone, nerve, ligament, organ, and gland. We observe the pulse of blood in our veins and the murmur of our nerves as they travel across fascia. We sense the weight of bone, the glide within joints, and the delicate motion of the cranial sutures. Moment by moment we attune to the flow of prana inside, inquiring, *How does it change? Where is it blocked? Is there irritation or ease?*

In meditation we similarly hone awareness so that sitting and breathing is, simply put, a practice in presence. In the early Buddhist teachings, the art of being present was defined in four foundations of mindfulness. The surge of mindfulness agendas that proliferate today in corporations, schools, health care clinics, and prisons stem from these four stages. The four foundations are a timeworn technology that, when installed in the yoga practitioner, lead to states of refined awareness. The stages of mindfulness are designed to cover the entire gamut of experience:

- Mindfulness of body and breath
- Mindfulness of sensation, feeling, and pulsation

- Mindfulness of thought, memory, attitude, and belief
- Mindfulness toward all phenomena, both outer and inner

In the practice of mindfulness, we orient to present time. In meditation it is easy to drift into another time zone—either into the past or into the future. You may find yourself rehashing a conversation that took place an hour ago or reliving an event that occurred a week, two weeks, or two years ago. Or you might be rehearsing what is to come, anticipating tonight's dinner or tomorrow's meeting. Whether rehashing or rehearsing, you lose touch with present time. There is nothing particularly wrong with mentally moving backward or forward in time—however, getting stuck there takes us out of the flow of presence. Like fish out of water, we get stranded in either the past or the future. Deprived of oxygen and the life that comes from immersion in the moment, our breath becomes shallow and we are ridden with anxiety and confusion. Disembodied, we get cut off from the very biological rhythms that sustain us—breath, heart rate, blood pressure, appetite, and the need for sleep. The vivifying spirit drains from us, and we lose touch with who we are.

Of the four foundations of mindfulness, I spend considerable time exploring the second stage, mindfulness of sensation. To be in the flow of presence, I "come back to my senses." When I am out of balance, like a boat that has tipped sideways, I set my keel down straight by bringing awareness to the sensations in my gut, the electrical pulses in my hands and feet, and the texture of my breath. By coming back to my senses, I locate myself smack-dab in the middle of where I am. Of all sensory experience, listening is paramount in yoga practice. Through the simple practice of listening—to ambient sounds in the environment or to the rhythm of the breath—it is possible to restore connection to present awareness. By coming back to our senses, we experience a kind of homecoming, a return to the very life force that sustains us.

In the beginning of our training, we practice diligently to arrive at the present moment. Yet in time we understand the present moment to be a slippery thing. If we investigate the present moment carefully, we realize that as soon as we think we have found it, the moment evaporates and is gone. Moments are fickle and evanescent. This is important, for over time we discover that there is no moment to capture. There is an expression in Zen: "seizing clouds, grasping at mist." We may try with all our might, but there is really no moment to grasp.

When we know there is nothing to grasp and there is no moment to "get," we feel lighter and more carefree. What happens when we stop attempting to grasp the moment? It is as if a heavy burden has been lifted off our shoulders. We are simply in the flow of presence, carried by an ever-rolling stream, that lifts us up and transports us. This well-known passage from the Diamond Sutra speaks elegantly to the transient now:

So you should see [view] all of the fleeting world:
A star at dawn, a bubble in the stream;

A flash of lightening in a summer cloud;

A flickering lamp, a phantom, and a dream.[4]

In practice we see that we and everything around us are constantly "under the law of change": weather patterns, political systems, technology, the pulse of blood through our veins, and our relationships with our loved ones. To be in the flow requires riding the edge of constant change.

Living on the cusp of transformation is the prerogative of the artist. All too often, we are reluctant to depart from familiar routines and we default to old habits to get by. This can narrow our perceptual field and stifle creativity. The music composer, artist, and Zen practitioner John Cage once said, "I can't understand why people are frightened of new ideas. I'm frightened of the old ones."[5] Each of us gets stuck in repetitive ways of thinking and behaving; the habit-mind can be like a snare, endlessly rehashing or rehearsing. We must be limber, adaptable, and agile to stay in the flow. In realizing that nothing is static or fixed (especially notions about self-identity), we can rise up to meet the demands of an ever-changing world.

Developing trust in the midst of uncertainty is challenging. Where can we find the faith to persevere? We develop trust by remembering that the present is right in front of our noses, always available. We need not go to India, refrain from eating, or push ourselves to the brink of exhaustion in order to realize this. It is always near, much closer than we ever could have imagined.

"Without realizing how near the truth is, we seek it far away," taught the Japanese Zen master Hakuin.

In the first years of my practice, I thought that present-moment awareness involved a heightened state of being. I always imagined awakening to be exotic, a transcendent state of super consciousness. I harbored a highfalutin' idea that yoga required achieving a mystical, sublime faculty. As a result, no matter what circumstance I found myself in, I assumed that it was not the magical and wondrous state of enlightenment. How could driving in traffic, taking out the trash, or discussing finances with my spouse be liberating?

Interested in capturing present-moment awareness in his art, John Cage reflected further on the importance of being in the now: "It is not irritating to be where one is. It is only irritating to think one would like to be somewhere else."[6] When Cage was composing music in the 1940s and 1950s, he was most drawn to creating scores that transported his audience to present-moment awareness. His novel piece 4′33″ was an experiment in immediacy, inviting audience members into the here and now. The score was four minutes and thirty-three seconds of silence. During the piece what emerged was the backdrop, the vast expanse of silence behind all sound. As with meditation, the "music" was stillness and silence and any momentary spontaneous ambient sounds—coughs, feet shuffling, a passing siren—became part of the composition.

The path of practice is to be with whatever arises and to remember that it is presenting itself to us with each step. It is not that we must get to the top of the proverbial mountain to realize present-moment awareness. Each and every step along the way is a manifestation of presence. The Chan master Yuanwu, who compiled and organized the Zen classic *The Blue Cliff Record* in China in 1112, described the path itself as a process of ongoing realization: "The bright road that the ancestors knew / is right in front of you, / in everything you see and hear."[7] How might we come to recognize that the experience of now is always right under our feet?

I like to consider the following three essential components to living in the now: intimacy, immediacy, and spontaneity. The first, intimacy, suggests close examination and attentive listening. The spirit of intimacy makes us receptive, sentient, and able to attend to the moment at hand. In every breath, every shift in bone, every passing train of thought, we develop intimacy. Without intimacy, a practice becomes oblivious and robotic. By necessity, intimacy involves proximity. Like a heart surgeon inserting a camera probe into the cardiac tissue to detect blockages in the ventricles, we learn to navigate the depths of experience with intricacy and finesse.

This is important because much of our time is spent at a distance: online learning, social media posts, and LinkedIn networking all involve remote communication. In the wireless era, people are connected but aloof, linked but isolated. Sherry Turkle, in her book *Alone Together*, suggests that our technologies create a divide on the most basic levels of intimacy, trust, honesty, and human connection. Devices make it *seem* that we are closer than ever before. I certainly feel this way when I phone my brother Michael, who lives in Bangalore, South India, and the connection on WhatsApp takes as long as it does for me to holler to my son upstairs in his bedroom. In the near future, much of our social interaction will be mediated by the cool touch of technology, as robotics and virtual reality become pervasive.

When we foster intimacy, we promote the free flow of awareness inside. When awareness is blocked or thwarted, it may result in numbing, constriction, and a lack of responsiveness in the bodily tissues. Thomas Hanna, a pioneer in somatic awareness and a senior student of Moshé Feldenkrais, coined the term "sensory-motor amnesia" to describe the vacant detachment that occurs when neurological and circulatory flow are cut off. To counter sensory-motor amnesia, we build somatic intelligence by opening the inner eye of perception. In somatic psychology, a capacity to perceive internally is called interoception. This involves "seeing within," a practice that has been a hallmark of meditative training since the earliest yoga practices. The Sanskrit word *vipassana* suggests this. *Vi* means "inside," and *pash* is the verbal root "to see." Inner seeing or interoception is an antidote to the ways in which we dissociate from our bodies.

Intimacy implies nonjudgmental presence. Without kindness, care, and patience, it is all too easy to become reactive. Intimacy demands that we pay close attention not only to pleasant states but also to feelings of anxiety, irritation, and pain. If we can acknowledge our pain without rejecting it or clinging to it, then we can learn to love. In this light, intimacy is the very root of nonharming (*ahimsa*).

Intimacy implies not only attending to the ecology of bodily sensation but also paying close attention to thoughts, attitudes, and emotions. If we sustain intimate connection, we can avoid spiraling into states of gloom and doom. When corrosive moods, thoughts, or beliefs arise, they can metastasize quickly through the body impacting respiration, digestive function, metabolic flow, and hormonal rhythms. Without a sense of intimacy, it is as if we are under a spell, possessed by forces outside ourselves. Often this leads to feelings of helplessness and a loss of personal power. Intimacy is typically associated with sex in our society; yet, ironically, sex is all too often devoid of intimacy, as it is driven by a need to control or to please. A practice that nurtures refined sensibility toward breath, sensation, and pulsation enables more conscientious connection in relationship.

The next valuable attribute to present-moment awareness is immediacy. Immediacy involves landing with both feet in the here and now. This helps to establish a sense of connection and belonging. Barbara Kingsolver draws a portrait of the reclamation of self through immediacy in her essay "High Tide in Tucson":

In my own worst seasons I've come back from the colorless world of despair by forcing myself to look hard, for a long time, at a single glorious thing: a flame of red geranium outside my bedroom window. And then another: my daughter in a yellow dress. And another: the perfect outline of a full, dark sphere behind the crescent moon.

Until I learned to be in love with my life again. Like a stroke victim retraining new parts of the brain to grasp lost skills, I have taught myself joy, over and over again.[8]

While classical yoga suggests detaching from sensory stimuli to concentrate the mind, it is valuable to be with what is happening now in order to mend broken sensory-motor connections. When there is numbness or rupture in the sensory-motor feedback loop, it is curative to "look hard for a very long time at a single thing." While sensory withdrawal (called *pratyahara*) is a key component in classical yoga, its corollary, sensory acuity, or sensory focusing, draws people to the present moment. As part of my teaching, I guide students through SATYA (Sensory Awareness for Yoga Attunement) practices. I invite students to hone their sensory awareness by directly perceiving their internal pulses. In this practice, we distill mindfulness down to the smallest of stimuli—the sound of a mourning dove outside the window, the trail of nerve impulses across the hip, the stretch of the skin at the back of the neck. By tracking the nuance of sensory experience, we turn the lantern of awareness back inside so that attention becomes more lucid and clear.

It is difficult to stay present when we are plagued by confusion and delusion. When confusion sends us into a tailspin, it can be curative to perform immediate, hands-on tasks. This might involve digging the dirt while gardening, knitting a sweater, or setting up a tent for the night. By engaging our sensory-motor awareness, we return to the ground of immediacy. By "chopping wood and carrying water," we come into the flow of presence. When I become caught up in my head and distracted, I spend time in my home landscape, placing native stones in the garden. While working with the texture, weight, shape, and color of rock, I am called back to a simple presence of being.

We come to immediacy through candid, straightforward experience. I am reminded of a verse by the Zen monk Koha:

> I cast the brush aside—
> from here on I'll speak to the moon
> face to face.[9]

All too often someone or something mediates our experience, and many times it is a screen. Given that our technologies are devoid of scent, texture, taste, or temperature, are we now further removed from contact with the moon? How can we put aside our media machines in order to "speak to the moon face to face"?

While at the beginning of practice we rely on techniques, protocol, and formula, at some point we must "cast the brush aside." This leads to intimate connection with the moment at hand.

The last of the three qualities that embody presence is spontaneity. We do not typically think of spontaneity as central to practice. It is likely that we have practiced with measured control—control of the body posture, the breath, and the mind. Yet it is through spontaneity that we connect to a raw, potent, unfiltered force—something more vast and powerful than ourselves. It is through spontaneity that the river of the Tao flows through us.

Allowing spontaneity into our lives can be challenging, especially if we have spent forty-five years in a schedule, micromanaging every day, week, and month. Typically, we do everything in our power to keep life on its chosen course. We live according to plan. However, when we succumb to orderly routine, we risk becoming islands of self-control. Excess control steals from the spirit and leaves us hollow but efficient. By giving ourselves permission to be spontaneous, we can experiment and be playful, open to both surprise and disappointment. Spontaneity always involves an element of risk. Children who are yet to manipulate themselves and their surroundings experience both the joy and the anguish that comes from spontaneity.

For most people, the fear of failure hamstrings both psychological and spiritual growth. As we age, we adhere to programmed, domesticated routines. "As our eyes grow accustomed to sight, they armor themselves against wonder," wrote the singer-songwriter Leonard Cohen. Spontaneity allows us to connect to wonder and the unpredictable ways that spirit moves.

In time we see that everything occurs on the spur of the moment. While there may be years of planning and rehearsal, nevertheless the moment arises "out of nowhere." This is the case as I write this book or when a movie director films a scene or when a mom sets boundaries for her child. We are actors on a great stage, delivering our lines extemporaneously. Each moment involves a tightrope walk between delivering from a set script and taking a step that we have never taken before. This is the raw beauty and fearful edge of being. As we give sanction to the spontaneous, our lives become less circumscribed and rote. The Tibetan mystic Shabkar, living high on the Himalayan plateau in northeast Tibet at the end of the eighteenth century, described the spontaneous flow of presence this way:

> Just as phenomena arise let them be and do not cling! This is the radical, essential practice during the daily round. . . . Its spontaneous manifestation of vivid appearances is a constant wonder. From the first to the last, the nature of all experience is pure! miraculously arisen! eternally free! completely free! effortlessly accomplished![10]

Relinquishing control in our lives is daunting. It poses an immediate threat to the ego's authority. While in the first half of practice we are eager to assume control over our diet, our bodies and thoughts, in the second phase of practice we are willing to relinquish the urge to engineer each and every experience.

This holds true for pranayama practice. Initially, I thought pranayama was the art of mastering the breath, guiding and manipulating its course. Many pranayama practices include ratio breathing in which the breath is divided numerically as in 5:10:10:5 (inhale for five seconds, retain for ten; exhale for ten seconds, retain for five). Measured breathing, however, imposes authority over the breath. In my own practice, I am most interested in supporting my prana to flow spontaneously of its own accord. In this way there is less of "me" invested in the practice. I am less interested in dominion over the breath and more inclined to let my breath flow through me uninhibited.

The question of control versus spontaneity is further illustrated by the function of the autonomic nervous system. The autonomic nervous system is the involuntary side of the nervous system and is outside of our conscious control. It is governed by smooth muscle and lines the windpipe, organs, and gut. On the other hand, the voluntary side of our nervous system is governed by striated muscle fibers—the ones that enable you to flex and extend your biceps or quads on command. Through postures like handstand and backbends, most yoga practices today emphasize the command side of the nervous system. But the autonomic nervous system governs our most essential life rhythms: heart rate, body temperature, breathing, digestion, sex drive, and appetite.

For millennia, yogis have sought to tap the wisdom of the autonomic nervous system. Its capacity to both animate and sustain life is ingenious. It is called the "inherent potency" in craniosacral work and is the underlying intelligence that governs all biological function. Its activity is regulated by structures installed deep in the brain stem and is likened to a reptilian force or serpent power (*kundalini*). Through fasting, not eating meat, not having sex, standing on their heads, or holding their breath, yogis have sought to vicariously regulate their autonomic nervous system and brainstem function. By identifying spontaneous shifts in breathing, blood pressure, body temperature, and nerve pulsation, we attune to an ancient and vital force. Critically, this life force is not our own, and it lies outside conscious control.

Thus it is through intimacy, immediacy, and spontaneity that we commune with the inherent potency. It is a primordial, elemental energy, a presence greater than ourselves, yet one that always includes us. It is both inside of us and all around us and is accessible in the smallest of gestures—a cloud, a memory, a breath. We need only remember that we are always in the presence of this potency, right here and now.

PRACTICE, INQUIRY, AND REFLECTION

IN MEDITATION

Listening through Stethoscopes

This practice builds a quality of intimacy by listening through imaginary stethoscopes, acoustic enhancers used by doctors to listen to heartbeat, intestinal activity, or circulatory flow. Assume a comfortable seat so that your pelvis is supported, and your spine is upright. Close your eyes so that your eyelids lightly touch. Let your eyes be delicate, as if you could feel a snowflake fall onto the lashes of your eyes. Settle into the weight of your bones and be sturdy, as if you were going to remain sitting still for a thousand years. Bring a sense of intimacy to the stream of your breath. Sense the texture of your breath as it filters through the back of your nostrils, along your windpipe, and into your lungs. Notice if you favor the inhalation or exhalation—that is, which phase of your breath comes easier for you?

Sensitize the skin along the sides of your skull. In particular, soften the skin around your ears and draw your ears inside so that your listening becomes softer and more acute. Imagine multiple stethoscopes placed on your skin throughout your body. Through these imaginary stethoscopes, listen to the nuanced pulsations of your breath, heartbeat, and nerves. Listen for the inherent potency that enlivens all your tissues. Place several stethoscopes on the sides of your skull. Listen with intimacy to the micropulses inside your cranium. Imagine placing a scope at the apex of your skull in order to sense the expansion and contraction of your cranial bones. Then place a scope at the bridge of your nose. Sense the bones (palatine, ethmoid, and sphenoid) in your front skull as light as the wings of a dragonfly. Sense the weight, pressure, and thickness of the structures across your brow. This is the region of the "third eye," the mystical gate that opens inward to the subtle body.

Next bring awareness to the immediacy of your breath. Imagine placing multiple stethoscopes on your trunk: on your sternum, ribs, belly, and chest. Listen to the amplified sounds of the murmur of your cardiac rhythm, the pump of your arterial flow, and the tremor of electrical activity along your nerves. Note any percussive sensations in your body as you sit. Do the sensations feel light, compressed, sharp, or thick? Where in the inner landscape of your body do you feel the sensations? You will likely feel a cacophony of different sounds: humming, purring, gurgling, rumbling sounds.

Place the imaginary stethoscopes intuitively on any surface of your body.

Then note the spontaneous movement of your breath. Observe the split second as your in-breath spontaneously emerges from the end of your out-breath. Notice any spontaneous murmur, pulsation, tingle, ripple, or tremor that accompanies your breath. As you rest in the flow of presence, listen globally to the inherent motion of all your living tissues.

ON THE MAT

Walking in the Flow of Presence

This practice involves outdoor walking. Find an open stretch of ground where you can walk. Begin by standing with your feet hip-width apart and your knees slightly bent. At the soles of your feet, make firm contact with the ground. Imagine that your legs are like the sturdy trunks of a tree. Visualize your feet extending down below the earth's surface as a vast root system. At the same time, lift the back of your skull upward and visualize the crown of your head connecting to the sky.

Begin taking slow, small steps. Bring awareness to the changes in pressure at the soles of your feet and the shifting kinetic forces that travel up through the bones and joints of your legs. Take approximately ten steps forward and then turn back, covering the same distance. The fact that you are not going anywhere enables you to concentrate on the flow of presence. Note the small shift in weight with each step. As you walk, note nuanced changes in your breathing, connective tissues, joints, and bones. Allow your attention to absorb into the slow movement of your gait. Remind yourself that everything transpires "under the law of change."

Note any sounds that occur in the environment around you. Note the drone of a far off plane, footsteps on the stairs, or the distant sound of a child's voice. What comes onto the screen of your attention? Bring a quality of intimacy to each step, heightening connection to your auditory, tactile, and visual experience. Be aware of your immediate connection to the ground, your breath, and the walking motion. Note any spontaneous fluctuations within your walk. Also note any shifts within the environment such as a sudden gust of wind or change in temperature. Allow your walking to be less about control and more about fluidity and ease in the flow of presence.

OFF THE MAT

In the River of Time

In the course of your day, practice being in the flow of the Tao by imagining that you are part of a great river of time. See that all your appointments, all the people you encounter, and the tasks you undertake are part of a larger flow. This flow of the Tao exists not only today, this week, and this year, but has been in motion for ten thousand years. Rather than fighting against it, allow the current of time to take you. It may trickle and cause you to feel bored. It may be slow and serene such that you feel relaxed and tranquil. Or it may be turbulent like whitewater rapids that cause you to become disoriented, spun around like a whirlpool. It is possible that you are taken down under the current and come up gasping for air.

Whatever scenarios arise for you today, remember that you are in the flow of a great river, the flow of the Tao. Do not fight the current of your day but rather trust in its course. Place confidence in the fact that you are always in the flow of presence. Be the path of water, flowing here and ebbing there sometimes turning and redirecting backward and at other times rushing forward. As you move through the circumstances of your day be alert, responsive, and prepared. Trust that in the flow of presence you can adapt to the changing circumstances around you in any way necessary.

9

Why Savasana Is the
Most Important Pose

THIS FINAL CHAPTER is dedicated to the final pose of our practice, savasana. You will recall that we started with savasana in order to "empty before you begin"; now we return, full circle, back to the start, back to the ground, and the process of letting go. We sometimes practice savasana at the beginning of class, sometimes in the middle and at the end of practice, for as we will see, savasana is the most important pose.

Most people translate *savasana* as "corpse pose," I think this is misleading and does not capture the magnitude of the pose. The deep state of rest that savasana affords does not lead to decay and destruction of the physical body—rather the practice of it acts as a salve to regenerate living tissue. If there is a death associated with savasana, it is of another kind. It is death of the small, smug, narrow-minded self. In this sense, savasana is a symbolic death and occurs not on a physical plane but on a psychic one. This psychic transmutation is implied by the Sanskrit verbal root *sav*, which means "to transform or alter." In savasana what decomposes (or to use the language of cremation, "burns up") is the myopic, obsessive, ego-clinging self. What remains has always been of real interest to the yogi. This final chapter is about what is left *after* savasana. That is to say, the end of savasana is really the beginning of the journey.

Savasana and its corollary yoga nidra (yogic sleep) transport us out into unconfined space—a space that is not co-opted by the ego's preferences, but is vast, generous, and capacious. Yoking body and mind in savasana, we enter a terrain greater than ourselves, a vast landscape that has no ultimate boundary or edge. On this walk we see that each of us is just a speck, a short-lived, infinitesimal mote. Like an astronaut suspended in an infinite universe, we rest in boundless space. This space is everywhere, from the outermost galaxy light years away to the cells inside our spleen.

As we saw in the first chapter, savasana allows us to release to the ground and become like the earth. This experience is unique for while we build solidity and mass, we also absorb into space (*akasha*). Being of the ground and of the air is paradoxical. In the practice of savasana, we are both matter and spirit, form and formless. The liminal space of savasana is the meeting point of heaven and earth.

The direct experience of space gives way to a feeling that is vast and subtle. In the meditative traditions of North India and Tibet, the essential nature of the mind is likened to open sky and uncluttered space. For this reason, yogi mystics dwell in the Himalayan plateau, where foot trails are etched across vast sweeps of mountain and the sky touches the ground. Proximity to the sky evokes a fathomless wonder, and yogis liken the essential nature of awareness to immeasurable space. Lama Shabkar, the venerated Dzogchen master wrote,

> By virtue of its all-penetrating freedom,
> This total presence has no center or circumference,
> No inside or outside,
> Is innocent of all partiality and
> Knows no blocks or barriers.
> This all-penetrating intrinsic awareness
> Is a vast expanse of space.
> All experience of samsara and nirvana
> Arise in it like rainbows in the sky.[1]

When awareness is as vast as space, it is a source of utmost serenity and peace. Space itself is likened to an experience of the nondual, for space is neither male nor female, black or white. It is not gay or straight, Republican or Democrat, Shiite or Suni, Protestant or Catholic, atheist or devout. Space "is innocent of all partiality." It has no center, no essence or truth.

The project of yoga is to embody a limitless, "total presence." Ironically, to do this, there must be a death. What dies is the singular, divisive, one-sided, erroneous self. This is because the bandwidth of the ego's identity is inevitably narrow. Its processing power is limited, and it is incapable of seeing two seemingly opposite realities at the same time. The death of the narrow-minded self is hard to come by for no one oversees his own demise willingly, even if it is the death of that which causes daily anguish and suffering. It is only when we are not looking and not in control that we can break through to an "all-penetrating freedom" that "knows no blocks or barriers." Thus we need the repose of savasana to embody this profound letting go.

This is not an easy task, as the elaborate coding within the ego-processor is difficult to quit. We could liken self-identity to a computer program, one that you logged onto once upon a time and now are helpless to shut down. The downloaded program of self, installed so long ago that you cannot remember a time without its function, is now your default operating system. It stores your pictures, your memories, and your sensory data. It comes equipped with its own thought processor that can compute and manage thousands of bits of information a minute. What makes shutting down the program especially troublesome is its fantastic range of controls and functions: it can build, create, destroy, imagine, pretend, love, and hate.

Periodically the program of self crashes. We might lose a loved one, get fired from a job, or receive a terminal diagnosis. This causes confusion in the internal system and as a result, we get stuck circling in place. When the program of self crashes unexpectedly, files get lost, messages get jumbled, and operations freeze. Then it is necessary to quit by force. Under the threat of a system shutdown, we panic and scramble furiously to reboot. The program of self-identity will do everything in its power to reassume procedural control, for it has encoded strict measures for its own survival. It will perform any operation necessary to maintain its domain functioning. It takes years (some say many lifetimes) to be able to realize that we have been running an imported software all along. This is why daily savasana is important.

Akin to the analogy of the self as a downloaded application, the language of the Bhagavad Gita likens the self to a garment that is put on and worn for a period of time. In this regard, we are each clothed in an identity—that is, we assume a gender, a history, a personality, and a role in life. We each have a name, a face, a social security number, and an e-mail address. We have likes and dislikes and unique ways of thinking, feeling, and behaving. When Krishna is coaching Arjuna, standing at the back of the war chariot prior to battle in the Bhagavad Gita, he gives instruction on the ephemeral nature of the body and its personality:

> Like the way a man casts away worn out clothes
> And later puts on new ones,
> So the great soul casts away worn out bodies
> In order to put on new ones.[2]

It is not just happenstance that Arjuna learns yoga while on the front line of battle. In the face of death, existential questions regarding karma, belief, and life's purpose become magnified. Not only does Arjuna have an opportunity to witness the evanescence of life by witnessing bodies being "cast away," but he is blessed to receive the illusive, grave, timeworn instructions on yoga. If the personality-identity and the body itself are like a cloak that is put on and taken off, the pressing question is this: *On what is the garment of self draped*? That is, what underlies the changeable, fashionable patterns in the shifting textile of self?

Considerable stretch is required to fathom the idea that the cloak of the presented self is an adornment. In today's fitness-crazed yoga, students are more intent on stretching hamstrings and hips and donning Lululemon than calling the personality-identity into question. Realizing that the life we wear is but a garment requires a deep stretch indeed. Arjuna, like all mortals, struggles to grasp the pivotal yoga teaching on the insubstantiality of self. And Arjuna has his own private yoga coach! Krishna is the archetypal support, literally standing at Arjuna's back in the war chariot and steering Arjuna through the myriad complex decisions of a lifetime. He counsels Arjuna to stretch beyond the confines of his own familial upbringing, beyond his professional duty, and beyond the assumptions he holds about the body in order to discern the nature of the great soul:

> Weapons cannot pierce it
> Fire does not burn it
> Water cannot wet it
> Nor can wind dry it out.
> This cannot be pierced, burned, moistened or withered;
> This is eternal, all pervading and unswerving
> It is imperturbable and primeval.[3]

The eternal and all-pervading source cannot be named or known with the interpretive mind or contacted through the sensory faculties. The best we can do is enter savasana and the sleep-like state of yoga nidra; they are thresholds to the inconceivable. Savasana then is a kind of bardo, suspended between two worlds—between sleep and wakefulness, death and rebirth. T. S. Eliot, himself a student of the Bhagavad Gita, famously wrote, "At the still point of the turning world. Neither flesh nor fleshless; / Neither from nor towards." Through repeated practices of savasana, the veil that separates the world of form from the realm of the formless appears flimsy. In savasana, we rehearse casting off the outer garb of self in order to rest at ease in the unadorned, naked space of awareness.

Biologically, savasana enables the regeneration of all bodily tissues. It is a panacea, helping to ward off all manner of sickness. In deep rest, the parasympathetic nervous system is activated to facilitate metabolic function: glandular rhythms reset, internal barometers governing blood pressure regulate, the heart rate slows, and intestinal activity increases.

For centuries, yogis have known the importance of sleep and have put into practice states that resemble sleep: seated meditation, savasana, and yoga nidra. It is well known today that sleep plays a significant role in repair and rejuvenation of both mind and body. Savasana is profoundly healing for it mimics the effects of sleep—it recalibrates the brain and central nervous system through a complex process of restoration. While the physiological benefits of sleep are important, yoga is most interested in its spiritual attributes. By absorbing into profound states of stillness, it is possible to rest in all pervading space. Residing in states that resemble sleep is comparable to putting your computer to sleep. If you leave your computer on with multiple programs running, your battery loses its charge.

Unfortunately, many people do not sleep well and as a result, lose their vital charge. Approximately one out of every nine people suffers from insomnia in America. This amounts to 40 million people. In his book *Why We Sleep*, Matthew Walker suggests that two out of three people have difficulty falling asleep or remaining asleep during the course of a single night.[4] Multiple factors may contribute to sleeplessness, including caffeine intake, excess ambient light in the bedroom, outside noise, imbalanced diet, and room temperature. Yet the primary causes of insomnia are often psychological—anxiety and emotional stress.

In savasana, awareness is meant to soak inside, so that all physiological function goes into deep relaxation. Like watering a tree down to its roots, meditation, savasana, and yoga nidra soak the very ground of being. Breath by breath, sensation by sensation, as the body relaxes and settles, a total suffusion of awareness penetrates all the cells. Like internal baptism, savasana bathes all the tissues, including the brain and spinal cord. Bathing and soaking practices are preparatory for the yoga state of samadhi.

It is important to note that sleep is not the absence of awareness. Awareness continues during sleep and may manifest in the guise of dreams, muscular activity, respiratory changes, speech, and so on. Multiple passages in the Upanishads celebrate connection to the unbroken thread of awareness woven through sleep and dream states. For example,

> In the state of deep sleep he does not see.
> Yet he is still knowing, for there is no cessation of the
> Knowing of the knower, because it is imperishable.[5]

In savasana we are meant to rest in the lucid awareness of the "knower." In the repose of savasana and yoga nidra, we develop a distilled, relaxed, and crystalline awareness. Classical yoga maps four states of consciousness: (1) waking, (2) sleep with dreaming, (3) sleep without dreaming, and (4) a most bare-bones, essential awareness referred to simply as "the auspicious" (*sivam*) or the "fourth" (*turiya*).

Earlier we explored how mindfulness is used to train awareness in the waking state of consciousness. In the second category of consciousness, sleep with dreaming, it is possible to trace the pathway of emotion and psychic content in the unconscious through dreamwork (see page 120). In this way, we enter the imaginative realm. Dream analysis was central to the birth of psychology in the West and both Freud and Jung investigated dreams to chart the interior psyche. Dreams are an amalgam of many complex forces, including autobiographical memory, sensory processing, hallucinogenic imagery, light display, motor movement, and emotional processing. In yoga, dreams have been used for years as tools for gaining insight and clarity in meditation. Sleep with dreaming is also known as rapid eye movement (REM), in which erratic flashings occur in the neural circuitry of the brain.

The third stage of consciousness, sleep without dreaming, is called non-REM (NREM) sleep. In this stage, brain activity is reduced and deep quiet prevails; flittering dream images are suspended while the brain's electrical waves become slow and regular. In NREM, brain waves synchronize in a profound electrical harmony. Like the way that breath halts or hovers in pranayama, respiration may suspend for a time in NREM sleep. If we imagine sleep to be like a slide projector, then the alternating slide images projected onto the screen are like dream displays in REM sleep. In NREM sleep the screen is blank except for the projected light from the projector's lumens.

In yoga, the fourth state of consciousness is described as "without distinctive marks," "unnamable," and "tranquil." In the analogy of the projector, it resembles the source of the light itself, irrespective of the screen.

At the outset of savasana training, the novice student will nod off to sleep or go out cold. At the end of class, in the yoga studio, you may recall hearing the gasps and sighs of someone snoring away in savasana. There is nothing wrong with this, and I believe that there is value in people resting or napping together in the same room. By participating in communal savasana, we move from the strict confines of individual consciousness to the shared space of a collective subconscious. Yet in savasana and its corollary, yoga nidra, we are meant to yoke to the boundless source that is everything. When there is complete relaxation of the body coupled with luminous, transparent awareness, we rest in the unitive state. The twelfth-century Chinese Chan master Hongzhi described it this way:

> Vast and spacious, like sky and water merging during autumn, like snow and moon having the same color, this field is without boundary, beyond direction, magnificently one entity without edge or seam. Further, when you turn within and drop off everything completely, realization occurs.[6]

Through savasana and meditation, we see that the construction of self is like a house of cards. It is tottery, precariously constructed, and hollow. We spend our growing years cobbling the ego together and with sufficient support (from family, peers, teachers, and coaches), the scaffolding of self gets established. However, the construction is rickety, makeshift. We cling to the insubstantial construct of self because it is short-lived. In the face of its own frailty, it girds itself in attempt to secure its own survival. When under threat, it assumes power and dominion over others or seeks control over its environment. Bound by the confines of its own construction, the small-minded self stays standing, unaware of a boundless potential just beyond its limited reach.

In the practice of savasana or meditation, the house of cards falls. I like to think of this giving way as the art of dropping. The process is astonishing and opens up an entirely new realm of possibility. Looking back, we realize how much energy we invested in simply keeping the structure of self intact. Until we see beyond the confines of our own limited selves, we fret and worry, fearful to lose what we have built. In any spiritual quest, this fear constrains maturation on the path. Fear is adhesive, like screws in the scaffolding, holding fast the small self to a seemingly solid structure.

When I was a twenty-something and in the early days of practice, I read Carlos Castaneda's tales about his escapades into the Sonoran Desert to learn the way of "seeing" from the native shaman Don Juan. Castaneda, the timid, overly intellectual anthropologist, eager to catch a glimpse of the other side, struggles to see beyond the confines of his own academic training. Castaneda undertakes an apprenticeship in native sorcery and is urged to see beyond the limits of his anxious, neurotic self:

> "The thing to do when you're impatient," he [Don Juan] proceeded, "is to turn to your left and ask advice from your death. An immense amount of pettiness is dropped if your death makes a gesture to you, or if you catch a glimpse of it, or if you just have the feeling that your companion is there watching you."[7]

We all suffer from petty-mindedness. We are prone to restless, myopic, and frivolous thinking. The path of the spiritual warrior necessitates the death of the trivial, narcissistic, ingrown self. We do not fully incarnate into the body of wisdom until this death occurs.

Many who survive near-death experiences attest to the way such an experience magnifies the preciousness of life and heightens appreciation for everyday living. In this sense, death is a guide, a guru. There is a poignant story told in the Katha Upanishad about a young man who gets sentenced to death in order to realize the teaching of yoga. Yama, the deity of death (literally the Great Restrainer), imparts the elusive, incomprehensible teachings on yoga. Yama shows how to die while living—a most difficult and perplexing task.

In savasana, when we drop to the ground and rest on the horizontal, we die while living, if only for a short time. Of course, we cannot exactly perceive this state or identify it in any way. If it could be seen or grasped, then someone would surely put it on the home page of their website and sell it for $99.99!

In the death of the myopic "me" in the second half of our journey, we no longer seek the approval of others or look to make more money, achieve more status, do more poses, get more Instagram followers, become enlightened, or make ourselves better.

In savasana we get stripped down to nothing. In spiritual training the process of leaving this world replicates entry into the world. When we leave the world, we are totally vulnerable, like a babe—beyond the senses, unclothed, raw, and tender. Savasana is a guide between worlds, through the sheer veil that hangs between life and death. When we practice savasana fifty times, one hundred times, ten thousand times, the veil between the two worlds becomes thinner, more transparent. Like the liminal state of bardo, savasana is a doorway, a portal from one side to the other. Through its practice we see that birth and death are but a continuum and that there really are no "sides." "Birth and death are the everyday practice of the Buddhist way," wrote Zen master Dōgen. Thus, at the end of savasana, we slowly roll to the side and swing up to sitting, head last. We roll up our mat and then move wholeheartedly into the flow of our day.

PRACTICE, INQUIRY, AND REFLECTION

IN MEDITATION

Sky Mind

Practice seated meditation directly after savasana. Sit comfortably so that your pelvis is propped upward and your spine is vertical. Allow the weight of your pelvic bones to settle and the weight of your upper legs to sink downward toward the floor. Imagine your upper legs to be made of wet sand so that your leg bones and sitting bones weigh downward. Like a tree growing toward the light, reach the base of your spine upward. Visualize space between your vertebrae in such a way that your intervertebral discs are buoyant. Be sure to lift the base of your cranium upward from the pedestal of your first cervical vertebra (C1). Simultaneously lower the front of your skull, without moving your head forward in space. Soften your eyes downward. Relax the skin on the sides of your skull while softening the cartilaginous tissue flaps around your ears. Imagine that you are in a deep state of sleep.

Practice savasana while seated. Allow the lightness and space you experienced in savasana on your back to pervade your entire body. This is the pose of the arch yogi Siva (*sivasana*). Make your breath very soft so that it becomes like the slightest of breezes. Sense your entire skull suffused with space. Allow a feeling of spaciousness to permeate your brain: behind your eyes, inside your middle ears, and throughout your back brain. Allow your awareness to become super fine and delicate. Like a vast open sky, imagine a boundless expanse of space filling every cell in your body. As you mimic the sleep state, let your awareness be clear, like the first light of dawn, soft like the sheen of a pearl. Fill your entire being with light and space.

ON THE MAT

Savasana: Between Waking and Sleeping

Lie on your back in savasana. As you lie down, elongate your spine from your sacrum to the crown of your head. Support your head with a blanket so that the back of your neck lengthens and there is no compression at the base of your skull. Place a rolled blanket or bolster underneath your knees so your sacrum can release into the floor. Place two to three blankets over your body so you are covered from your neck to your feet. If you have a sandbag, place it atop your pelvis. Sense how the cover and weight allow you to "cocoon" into the pose.

Feel the weight of your body drop and widen. Let your breath become very soft, shallow, and slow. Your breath should slow to such a degree that you almost stop breathing. With each breath and with each passing moment, draw your awareness inside. Observe how your awareness soaks inward. Seep down into the ground like water poured into dry earth. Visualize the weight of the back of your skull widening and spreading out on the floor. Be sure that your eyes soften and sink toward the back of your skull. With each exhalation, sense the cells in the frontal lobes of your brain, releasing backward toward the floor. At the same time, note the feeling of lightness at your forehead. Imagine that the bone of your forehead (frontal bone) floats upward toward the ceiling enabling a profound relaxation to penetrate the nerve cells of your forebrain. Sense the way that your awareness hovers between waking and sleep. Be like mist hanging over a lake in the early hours at dawn.

Suspend in this state of stillness and repose while allowing deep relaxation to diffuse throughout your entire body. Rest for fifteen minutes before rolling to your side to come up.

OFF THE MAT

Reflections on Death

In the Parinirvana Sutra, composed around the second century, it is said, "Of all meditations, that on death is supreme." At the end of the path we pause and consider: What it is like to die? Hopefully, at the culmination of life we still have our wits about us, but that is a big *if.* Many die in a stupor, either throttled by dementia, in a blue haze of morphine, or in a swoon of confusion. If at all possible, we are mindful to the end. But death is as unpredictable as life.

We don't know if death will come in the day or the night, as a slow fade or a flash. The body has no built-in expiration date. Generally, life is like a locomotive that churns and pushes across mountains, valleys, and open plains. We never imagine it coming to a halt. Until it does.

Perhaps you have had the opportunity, bedside, to be with someone as they enter the tunnel of death. It is a gift to witness the flame of life flickering and fading. All petty concerns, all gripes and grudges drop away. Death is the great equalizer. It is both raw and beautiful to witness. Death moves in its own time capsule— moments hang suspended like stars in far-off galaxies. There is nothing to do about death. You may offer encouragement, saying, "It's all right, you can let go." But the letting go must begin much earlier. The lesson of letting go cannot be realized in the fleeting moments as the breath leaves the body. This is why savasana is so important. Savasana is the dress rehearsal for death, so that if possible, we remember in our cells, our diaphragm, our heart and mind, how to let go.

The process of dying is a plunge into mystery where being with not knowing is the most we can do. It is an irony that we spend most of our day making sense, figuring things out. In the practice of savasana and on death's doormat, there is no further calculation. In the throes of dying, reason loses traction. You have to just be with what is.

At death's door there is a kind of cocooning. It is as if the dying are inside a chrysalis, incubating. Unable to see, taste, or touch, the pupa's innards are soft, raw, and vulnerable. In this way death is like birth. There is a period of gestation when the animating spirit tucks into itself, preparing to shape-shift and move on. Savasana, too, involves a process of cocooning. In savasana we are swaddled, folded inward so that we may rest deeply. We may use blankets, eye pillows, or sandbags to coax the life force to retreat far inside. In savasana the prana submerges and returns home, back to the source from which it came.

At the end of life, a force kicks in that is beyond reckoning. It's as old as the coelacanth, as astounding as the tiger, and as immeasurable as the stars. At the very end there is nothing but breath and the strange alchemy of prana. It moves of its own accord, propelled by the Great Regulator, far down the brainstem.

We visualize the final transition. It is a passage, like entry through the birth canal or a slow descent down a spiral staircase. It is like the custom of the Native American tribes of the Northwest who transport their dead by placing the body in a canoe and floating it downriver to catch the ebbing tide out to sea.

Notes

1. EMPTY BEFORE YOU BEGIN

1. Yoel Hoffman, *Japanese Death Poems: Written by Zen Monks and Haiku Poets on the Verge of Death* (Boston, Tuttle Publishing, 1986), 303–304.
2. Tias Little. *The Bhagavadgita*, chap. 6, verses 24–25.
3. David Ignatow, "Content," in *Against the Evidence: Selected Poems, 1934–1994* (Middletown, CT: Wesleyan University Press, 1994), 45.
4. Thomas Merton, *The Asian Journal of Thomas Merton* (New York: New Directions Publishing, 1975), 117.
5. Heinrich Robert Zimmer, *Myths and Symbols in Indian Art and Civilization* (Princeton, NJ: Princeton University Press, 2015), 44.

2. ALWAYS NEW

1. Bhikkhu Ñāṇamoli and Bhikku Bodhi, *The Middle Length Discourses of the Buddha: A Translation of the Majjhima Nikāya* (Boston, MA: Wisdom Publications, 1995), 229.

2. Juan Ramón Jiménez, "Oceans," *News of the Universe, Poems of Twofold Consciousness*, trans. Robert Bly (San Francisco, Sierra Club Books, 1980), 105.

3. Marcel Proust, *In Search of Lost Time*, trans. Lydia Davis (London: Penguin Books, 2003).

3. HOW SPEED GETS TRAPPED IN THE BODY

1. Thomas Merton, *New Seeds of Contemplation* (New York: New Directions, 2007), 98–99.

2. Pico Iyer and Eydís Einarsdóttir, *The Art of Stillness: Adventures in Going Nowhere* (New York: TED Books/Simon & Schuster, 2014), 66.

3. Lao-Tzu, *Lao-Tzu Te-Tao Ching*, trans. Robert G. Henricks (New York, Ballantine Books, 1989), 192.

4. Rollo May, *Love & Will* (New York: Norton, 2007), 15.

5. THE QUEST FOR THE PERFECT POSE

1. Tias Little, *The Heart Sutra*, lines 10–11.

2. Ikkyu, "Crow with No Mouth," *Ikkyu: Fifteenth Century Zen Master*, trans. Stephen Berg (Port Townsend, WA: Copper Canyon Press, 2000), 26.

3. Leonard Cohen, *The Future*, Columbia Records, 1992, CD.

6. NOT KNOWING

1. Thich Nhat Hanh, *The Heart of Understanding* (Berkeley, CA: Parallax Press, 1988), 24.

2. Natalie Goldberg, *Old Friend from Far Away* (New York: Atria, 2007), 242.

3. Bernie Glassman, *Bearing Witness: A Zen Master's Lessons in Making Peace* (New York: Belltower, 1998), 27.

4. *Lion's Roar* staff, "Why Bernie Glassman keeps going back to Auschwitz," *Lion's Roar*, March 12, 2013. www.lionsroar.com/why-bernie-glassman-keeps-going-back-to-auschwitz/.

5. Walt Whitman, "Song of the Open Road," *The Complete Poems* (New York: Penguin Books, 1975), 181.

6. Tias Little. *Mandukya Upanishad*. Verse 7.

7. Andrew Brook, *Kant and the Mind* (Cambridge: Cambridge University Press, 1997), 247.

8. Kenneth Cohen, *The Way of Qigong* (New York: Random House, 2018), 137.

9. Lama Mipham, *Calm and Clear* (Berkeley: Dharma Publishing 1973), 46.

7. THE OM SHANTI EXPERIENCE

1. C. G. Jung, *The Psychology of Kundalini Yoga* (Princeton, NJ: Princeton University Press, 1996), xxv.

2. Wendell Berry, "To Know the Dark," *Farming: A Handbook* (Berkeley: Counterpoint, 2011), 26.

3. Matsuo Basho, *Zen Poetry* trans. Lucien Stryk and Takashi Ikemoto (London, England. Penguin Books 1977), 87.

4. Peter Levine, *Waking the Tiger* (Berkeley, CA: North Atlantic Books, 1997), 12.

5. Jane Hirshfield, "A Cedary Fragrance," *Given Sugar, Given Salt* (New York: HarperCollins, 2001), 32.

8. IN THE FLOW OF PRESENCE

1. Alan Watts, *Tao: The Watercourse Way* (New York: Pantheon Books, 1975), 47.

2. Watts, *Tao*, 37.

3. Watts, *Tao*, 45.

4. Mu Soeng, *The Diamond Sutra* (Boston: Wisdom Publications, 2000), 135.

5. Richard Kostelanetz, *Conversing with Cage* (New York: Routledge Press, 2003), 221.

6. John Cage, "Lecture on Nothing," in *Silence: Lectures and Writings, 50th Anniversary Edition* (Middletown, CT: Wesleyan University Press 2013), 119.

7. Joan Sutherland, *Acequias and Gates*, (Santa Fe, NM: Following Wind Press, 2013), 25.

8. Barbara Kingsolver, *High Tide in Tucson* (New York: HarperCollins, 1995), 15.

9. Hoffman, *Japanese Death* Poems, 229.

10. Keith Dowman, *The Flight of the Garuda: The Dzogchen Tradition of Tibetan Buddhism* (Somerville, MA: Wisdom Publications, 2003), 96–97.

9. WHY SAVASANA IS THE MOST IMPORTANT POSE

1. Dowman, *Flight of the Garuda*, 76. Used by permission.

2. Little. *Bhagavad Gita*. chap. 2, verse 22.

3. Little, *Bhagavad Gita*, chap. 2, verse 24.

4. Matthew Walker, *Why We Sleep: Unlocking the Power of Sleep and Dreams* (New York: Simon and Schuster, 2018), 265.

5. Little, *Brhadaranyaka Upanishad*, chap. 4, verse 23.

6. Taigen Daniel Leighton with Yi Wu, *Cultivating the Empty Field: The Silent Illumination of Zen Master Hongzhi*, (San Francisco, CA: North Point Press, 1991), 8–9.

7. Carlos Castaneda, *Journey to Ixtlan* (New York: Simon and Schuster, 1972), 34.

References

Berry, Wendell. *Farming: A Handbook*. Berkeley: Counterpoint, 2011.

Bhikkhu Ñāṇamoli, trans. *The Middle Length Discourses of the Buddha: A Translation of the Majjhima Nikāya*. Translation edited and revised by Bhikkhu Bodhi. Boston: Wisdom Publications, 1995.

Bly, Robert. *News of the Universe: Poems of Twofold Consciousness*. San Francisco, CA: Sierra Club Books, 1980.

Brook, Andrew. *Kant and the Mind*. Cambridge: Cambridge University Press, 1997.

Castaneda, Carlos. *The Teachings of Don Juan*. Berkeley, CA: University of California Press, 2016.

Cohen, Kenneth S. *The Way of Qigong*. New York: Random House International, 2013.

Cohen, Leonard. *The Future*. Columbia Records, 1992. CD.

Dowman, Keith. *The Flight of the Garuda: The Dzogchen Tradition of Tibetan Buddhism*. Somerville, MA: Wisdom Publications, 2014.

Glassman, Bernie. *Bearing Witness: A Zen Master's Lessons in Making Peace*. New York: Belltower, 1998.

Goldberg, Natalie. *Old Friend from Far Away*. New York, Atria Books, 2007.

Hanh, Thich Nhat. *The Heart of Understanding*. Berkeley, CA: Parallax Press, 1988.

Henricks, Robert G. *Lao-Tzu Te-Tao Ching*. New York: Ballantine Books, 1989.

Hirshfield, Jane. *Given Sugar, Given Salt*. New York: Perennial, 2002.

Hoffman, Yoel. *Japanese Death Poems*. Boston: Tuttle Publishing, 1986.

Ignatow, David. *Against the Evidence: Selected Poems, 1934–1994*. Middletown, CT: Wesleyan University Press, 1994.

Iyer, Pico, and Eydís Einarsdóttir. *The Art of Stillness: Adventures in Going Nowhere*. New York: TED Books/Simon & Schuster, 2014.

Jung, C. G. *The Psychology of Kundalini Yoga*. Princeton, NJ: Princeton University Press, 1996.

Kingsolver, Barbara. *High Tide in Tucson: Essays from Now or Never*. New York: Perennial, 2003.

Kostelanetz, Richard. *Conversing with Cage*. New York: Routledge Press, 2003.

Levine, Peter. *Waking the Tiger*. Berkeley: North Atlantic Books, 1997.

Machado, Antonio. *There Is No Road*. Translated by Mary G. Berg and Dennis Maloney. Buffalo, NY: White Pine Press, 2003.

May, Rollo. *Love & Will*. New York: Norton, 2007.

Merton, Thomas. *The Asian Journal of Thomas Merton*. New York: New Directions Publishing, 1975.

———. *New Seeds of Contemplation*. Boston: Shambhala Publications, 2003.

———. *The Other Side of the Mountain: The End of the Journey*. Edited by Patrick Hart. San Francisco: HarperOne, 1999.

Mipham, Lama. *Calm and Clear*. Berkeley: Dharma Publishing, 1973.

Pert, Candace B. *Molecules of Emotion*. New York: Scribner, 1997.

Shizutero, Uedo. *Bashō*. Tokyo: Iwanami Shoten, 2003.

Soeng, Mu. *The Diamond Sutra*. Boston: Wisdom Publications, 2000.

Sutherland, Joan. *Acequias and Gates: Miscellaneous Koans and Writings on Miscellaneous Koans.* Santa Fe, NM: Following Wind Press, 2013.

Stryk, Lucien, and Takashi Ikemoto. *Zen Poetry*. London: Penguin, 1977.

Turkle, Sherry. *Alone Together: Why We Expect More from Technology and Less from Each Other*. New York: Basic Books, 2017.

Walker, Matthew P. *Why We Sleep: Unlocking the Power of Sleep and Dreams*. New York: Simon & Schuster, 2018.

Watts, Alan, and Al Chung-liang Huang. *Tao: The Watercourse Way*. Harmondsworth, UK: Penguin Books, 1981.

Whitman, Walt. *The Complete Poems*. New York: Penguin Books, 1975.

Yuanwu. *The Blue Cliff Record*. Translated by Thomas F. Cleary and J. C. Cleary. Boston: Shambhala Publications, 2005.

Zhengjue. *Cultivating the Empty Field: The Silent Illumination of Zen Master Hongzhi*. Translated by Taigen Daniel Leighton with Yi Wu. Boston: Tuttle Publishing, 2000.

Zimmer, Heinrich. *Myths and Symbols in Indian Art and Civilization*. Edited by Joseph Campbell. Princeton, NJ: Princeton University Press, 2017.

About the Author

Tias Little synthesizes years of study in classical yoga, Sanskrit, Buddhism, and anatomical study in his dynamic, original style of teaching. Tias began studying the work of B. K. S. Iyengar in 1984 and in 1989 resided in Mysore, India, where he studied Ashtanga vinyasa yoga under the tutelage of Sri K. Pattabhi Jois.

A licensed massage therapist, Tias has in-depth training in craniosacral therapy. His practice and teaching is influenced by the work of Ida Rolf, Moshé Feldenkrais, and Thomas Hanna. He earned a master's degree in Eastern philosophy from St. John's College in Santa Fe in 1998. Tias is the founder of the Prajna Yoga school in Santa Fe, where he hosts retreats, workshops, and teacher-training programs year-round with his wife, Surya. Tias is the author of three books: *The Thread of Breath, Meditations on a Dewdrop* and *Yoga of the Subtle Body* (Shambhala, 2016) For more on Tias, visit www.prajnayoga.net.